BLOOD TYPE O DIET COOKBOOK FOR BEGINNERS

Easy-to-Follow Recipes and Vital Advice for Peak Health Customized to Your Blood Group

Tim Lingard

Table of Contents

Beef & Pork

As a token of our gratitude for your purchasing our book, we will be providing you with extra bonuses.

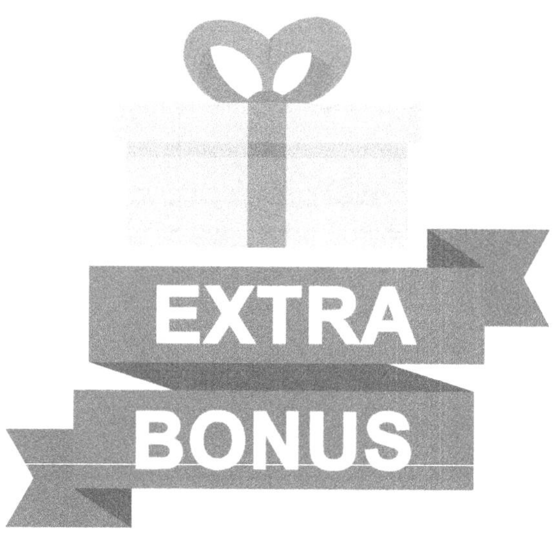

1. WEEKLY MEAL PLANNER JOURNAL
2. FREE E-BOOK featuring FULL-COLOR IMAGES OF THE FINISHED RECIPES.
3. A PRIVATE CONSULTATION SESSION

Special Note

It's important to remember that the path to wellness is as unique as you are. This cookbook is crafted to help you explore the profound connection between your blood type and your diet, offering recipes that are tailored to enhance the health and vitality of those with Type O blood.

However, the art of personal health is finely tuned to individual needs. While the guidance provided in this book is based on extensive research and has been tailored to suit the general characteristics of Type O individuals, it's essential to listen to your own body and adjust accordingly. You know yourself best—your tastes, your reactions, and your health goals. Feel empowered to tweak the recipes to better suit your specific dietary requirements and preferences.

We also encourage you to consult with a healthcare professional, especially if you find yourself unsure or if you have pre-existing health conditions. A dietitian or a doctor can offer invaluable insights and guidance, ensuring that the dietary changes you make are beneficial and in harmony with your overall health plan.

Please note that the nutritional information provided with each recipe is approximate. Variations in ingredient choices and preparation methods can affect the nutritional values. Whether you're substituting an ingredient or adjusting portion sizes, the nutritional impact may vary slightly from what is documented.

Furthermore, if this cookbook has enhanced your cooking and dining experience, we would love to read about your journey in an Amazon review. Conversely, if you encounter any issues with the recipes, please feel free to reach out to us at **timlingard98@gmail.com**. We are dedicated to assisting you throughout your culinary adventure.

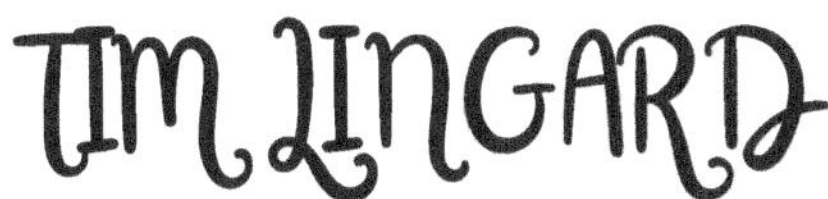

Introduction.

Welcome to a journey of transformation and well-being that is as delicious as it is healthful! As you turn these pages, you're not just opening a cookbook—you're stepping into a new way of understanding how your body interacts with the very essence of nourishment. There's more to **Blood Type O Diet Cookbook for Beginners** than just a list of meals; it's a personalized guide to eating that aligns with your unique genetic makeup.

If you are among the many with blood type O, you hold in your hands a blueprint to better health tailored specifically for your body's needs. The significance of eating according to your blood type cannot be overstated. As the most common, yet evolutionarily ancient of blood types, Type O carries with it the genetic memory of strength, endurance, and a robust immune system. However, in today's fast-paced world, maintaining a lifestyle that truly nurtures this genetic legacy can be challenging. This book is your ally in that endeavor. Why a diet book specifically for Type O? Because not all foods affect every individual in the same way. What energizes and heals one person might be ineffective or even harmful for another. The Blood Type O Diet focuses on how foods interact with your blood type at the cellular level, influencing your digestive system, immune response, and overall health. It is about making choices that enhance your well-being, reduce inflammation, and optimize your energy levels. It's about rediscovering the harmony of living in sync with your body's natural rhythms. Each recipe in this cookbook has been meticulously designed to cater to the Type O metabolism, which thrives on protein-rich foods like meat and fish while reacting sensitively to gluten and some legumes. But it's not just about eliminating what doesn't work—it's about embracing a plethora of ingredients that do. You'll find dishes that range from hearty breakfasts to satisfy your carnivorous side, to refreshing salads and sides that integrate foods beneficial to your type

.As you explore these pages, you'll encounter meals that speak directly to the soul of Type O—dishes that are simple yet bold, flavors that are robust and earthy. Imagine starting your day with a vibrant Berry and Flaxseed Smoothie or sitting down to a dinner of Roasted Lamb with Rosemary coupled with a side of Garlic Mashed Sweet Potatoes.

Picture ending your day with a satisfying and soothing Chamomile and Peppermint tea, knowing every sip and every bite is designed to make you feel your best. This cookbook is your gateway to understanding how deeply food influences our bodies and our lives. It invites you to experiment, to taste, and to feel the changes as your body responds to foods that are meant for you. Whether you're a seasoned chef or just beginning your culinary journey, these recipes are crafted to be accessible, with straightforward instructions and tips on how to incorporate the Blood Type O Diet into your everyday life.

Blood Type O Diet Cookbook for Beginners is not just about eating differently; it's about making a profound connection with your food. It's about the joy of cooking and the peace that comes from knowing you are truly nourishing yourself. So, embrace this journey with enthusiasm and curiosity. Allow this book to be a companion in your quest for a healthier, more vibrant you. Let's begin this flavorful adventure together!

Chapter 1

UNDERSTANDING YOUR BLOOD TYPE

The Basics of Blood Typing

Your blood type is determined by specific antigens present on the surface of your red blood cells. These antigens are essentially chemical markers that your body uses to recognize its own cells from foreign cells, an essential part of the immune response. There are four major blood types: A, B, AB, and O, each of which can be positive or negative based on the presence of the Rh factor, another type of antigen.

Blood Type O Characteristics

Blood Type O is often called the "universal donor" type for its compatibility in blood transfusions. This type lacks the A and B antigens found in other blood groups, making its red blood cells less likely to be rejected by a recipient's immune system. But beyond transfusions, the lack of these antigens has broader implications for health and well-being.

1. Diet and Digestion

People with Type O blood may digest meat well due to high levels of stomach acid, making them excellent at processing protein and fat. However, this can mean they might have more trouble digesting foods that are high in carbohydrates, like wheat and certain grains. Thus, a protein-rich diet is often recommended for those with Type O blood.

2. Immune System

The natural presence of certain antibodies makes Type O individuals less susceptible to some diseases, but more to others. For instance, they are generally at a lower risk for heart disease and blood clotting disorders but may be more vulnerable to ulcers due to high stomach acid levels.

3. Stress Response

The stress hormone, cortisol, tends to be higher in people with Type O blood. They might be more prone to anger or hyperactivity when stressed and might benefit greatly from regular, intense physical activity. Physical exercises not only help mitigate the stress response but also support overall vitality and health.

4. Personality Traits

Though scientific evidence is mixed, proponents of blood type diets suggest that those with Type O blood might tend to be assertive, practical, and organized, but on the flip side, they can also be more prone to anger, hyperactivity, and impulsiveness. Whether these observations have biological roots or are merely coincidental is still up for debate.

Why Does It Matter?
Knowing your blood type does more than prepare you for safe transfusions or understanding dietary needs. It's about tailoring lifestyle choices that optimize your health. For Type O individuals, this might mean adopting a specific diet, engaging in vigorous exercise, and developing effective stress-management techniques.

HEALTH BENEFITS OF THE BLOOD TYPE DIET

The Blood Type Diet, popularized by Dr. Peter J. D'Adamo in his book "Eat Right for Your Type," proposes that one's diet should be tailored according to one's blood type—A, B, AB, or O—to optimize health. This concept suggests that the foods you eat react chemically with your blood type, and if you follow a diet designed for your blood type, it can help improve health and decrease risk of chronic diseases. Let's examine some of the purported health benefits associated with this diet, focusing on what it might mean for people of different blood types.

1. Improved Digestive Health

One of the key benefits often cited by proponents of the Blood Type Diet is improved digestive health. According to the theory, each blood type has its own response to certain types of foods. For example:

- **Type O**: High in stomach acid, better suited to digesting proteins and fats. Therefore, a diet high in lean meats, poultry, and fish is beneficial, while grains, beans, and legumes might cause digestive issues.
- **Type A**: Lower stomach acid but a tolerant immune system, which makes a primarily vegetarian diet ideal for this group. Soy proteins, grains, and organic vegetables are encouraged.
- **Type B**: The only blood type that does well with dairy products. This group supposedly has a versatile digestion and can thrive on moderate amounts of meats, dairy, and grains.
- **Type AB**: Combines some aspects of both A and B types, often benefiting from a diet that includes seafood, tofu, dairy, and an array of vegetables.

By eating according to your blood type, the theory suggests you can improve your body's ability to digest and assimilate nutrients, thereby reducing gastrointestinal issues, such as bloating, gas, and indigestion.

2. Increased Energy Levels

Following a Blood Type Diet can purportedly lead to increased energy levels. This might be attributed to the removal of foods that cause an adverse chemical reaction in your body. For example, Type O's consuming less gluten-containing grains and more protein might experience a boost in energy as they avoid the energy slumps often associated with carbohydrate-heavy meals.

3. Weight Management

Many followers of the Blood Type Diet report easier weight management when adhering to the recommended eating plan for their type. This is thought to be due to the diet's emphasis on natural, whole foods over processed foods and tailored nutrient intake. For instance, the recommended diet for Type A emphasizes a plant-based diet, which is generally lower in calories and fats, potentially helping with weight loss or maintenance.

4. Reduced Risk of Diseases

Proponents argue that by following a Blood Type Diet, individuals can potentially reduce their risk of certain diseases. For Type O, which is associated with a robust digestive tract but a high predisposition to inflammation, eating lean meats and avoiding inflammatory grains can purportedly decrease the risk of metabolic syndrome, cardiovascular disease, and insulin resistance.

5. Better Overall Health

By eating foods that are genetically harmonious with your blood type, the diet claims to improve the immune system, helping to prevent viruses and infections. For example, Type B individuals who consume immune-boosting foods like greens, eggs, and certain types of meat may experience fewer bouts of disease and better overall health.

While the Blood Type Diet provides a structured food choice system that many find beneficial, it's important to note that scientific support for blood-specific diets is limited. The diet encourages a healthy intake of fruits, vegetables, and whole foods while limiting processed foods, which in itself is beneficial regardless of blood type. If you're considering this diet, it may be useful to first experiment with the recommended foods for your type to see if you notice improvements in digestion, energy, and general well-being. However, it's always best to consult with a healthcare provider before starting any new diet regimen to ensure it fits your individual health needs and goals.

THE BASICS OF THE BLOOD TYPE O DIET

For those who are new to the field of customized nutrition, the Blood Type O Diet presents a fascinating approach tailored to the most common blood type globally. This diet, based on the premise that your blood type can influence how your body interacts with certain foods, suggests that people with Type O blood may experience better health outcomes by following a specific eating pattern. Let's break down what this diet involves, why it might be beneficial, and how to implement it effectively.

Understanding Blood Type O

Blood Type O is often described as the oldest and most common blood type, associated historically with ancestors who were hunters and gatherers. This lineage suggests that individuals with this blood type might thrive on a diet similar to what those early humans ate—high in protein, low in carbohydrates, and rich in fruits and vegetables.

Key Dietary Focus for Type O

The cornerstone of the Blood Type O Diet is protein consumption from meat. High protein intake is emphasized because people with this blood type are thought to have high stomach-acid levels, which makes digesting animal protein easier. Here's a more detailed look at the dietary recommendations:

1. Protein Sources

- **Meat:** Beef, lamb, and venison are considered ideal for Type O individuals. These red meats are rich in the amino acids that Type O's reportedly metabolize well.
- **Poultry and Fish:** While chicken can be problematic for some Type O individuals due to an inflammatory response, other poultry like turkey is recommended. Fish, especially oily ones rich in omega-3 fatty acids like salmon and mackerel, are also beneficial.

2. Limited Grains and Legumes

- People with Type O blood are advised to limit grain and legume intake. Wheat and corn can contribute to weight gain and disrupt insulin regulation for Type O's. Instead, grains like rice and buckwheat, which are gluten-free, are better tolerated.
- Legumes can also interfere with digestion and nutrient absorption, with some like lentils and kidney beans being particularly problematic.

3. Fruits and Vegetables
- Fruits and vegetables are crucial for providing vitamins, minerals, and fiber. However, certain vegetables like Brussels sprouts, cabbage, and cauliflower are suggested to be avoided as they can inhibit thyroid function in Type O's.
- Beneficial fruits include plums, prunes, and figs, which help the digestive tract function properly and counteract the muscle tissue breakdown from the high protein intake.

4. Dairy and Eggs
- Dairy products are generally minimized in the Blood Type O Diet. Due to the presumed ancestral lack of dairy digestion, Type O individuals may be more prone to issues like bloating and inflammation from dairy.
- Eggs, on the other hand, can be a good protein source, although moderation is key.

5. Fats and Oils
- Healthy fats are essential. Olive oil and certain nut oils (like walnut) are good choices, providing necessary fats without the adverse effects associated with saturated fats found in some meats and dairy products.

Implementing the Diet

Adopting the Blood Type O Diet involves more than just choosing the right types of food; it's about adjusting your eating habits to maximize your body's natural metabolic processes. Here are a few tips:
- **Meal Planning:** Plan meals that balance protein with ample amounts of vegetables and a modest amount of fruits and fats.
- **Cooking Methods:** Opt for healthier cooking methods like grilling, broiling, or steaming rather than frying.
- **Listen to Your Body:** Everyone is unique, even within blood type categories. Pay attention to how your body reacts to changes in your diet and adjust accordingly.

Hence, the Blood Type O Diet encourages a return to the basics—favoring a high-protein, low-carbohydrate diet that may mimic the eating patterns of our hunter-gatherer ancestors. While scientific consensus on the effectiveness of blood type diets remains mixed, many find this approach helpful for digestion, energy levels, and overall health.

Foods to Embrace

Choosing the right foods can enhance your dietary experience, making it not only a nutritious journey but also a delightful exploration of flavors that are beneficial for your body. Here are some foods that are typically recommended for their health benefits and compatibility with specific dietary needs:

1. Lean Proteins

- For meat eaters, especially those on a Type O diet, lean meats such as turkey, lamb, and lean beef are ideal. These proteins are rich in iron and help increase metabolism.
- Fish, particularly cold-water fish like salmon and mackerel, is encouraged for its high omega-3 fatty acid content, which supports cardiovascular health and reduces inflammation.

2. Vegetables

- A wide array of vegetables should form the cornerstone of your diet. Leafy greens such as spinach, kale, and Swiss chard are packed with vitamins, minerals, and fiber, which aid digestion and support overall health.
- Other beneficial vegetables include broccoli, peppers, and carrots, which provide essential nutrients and antioxidants.

3. Fruits

- While fruit selection can vary by diet type, generally, fruits such as berries, apples, and pears are encouraged due to their high fiber and antioxidant properties.
- For those concerned with sugar intake, low glycemic fruits like cherries, plums, and grapefruit are excellent choices that provide flavor without spiking blood sugar levels.

4. Whole Grains

- Whole grains like quinoa, rice, and oats are excellent sources of fiber and keep you full longer. These grains are generally well tolerated and do not provoke the insulin response that refined grains might.

5. Healthy Fats

- Incorporating healthy fats into your diet is essential for maintaining good health. Avocados, nuts, seeds, and olive oil are not only delicious but also rich in fats that promote heart health and reduce harmful cholesterol levels.

Foods to Avoid

Just as important as knowing what to eat is understanding what foods to avoid. Certain foods can exacerbate health issues or detract from the benefits of a well-tailored diet:

1. Processed Foods
- Highly processed foods are universally recognized as detrimental to health. These include fast foods, high-sugar snacks, and anything with artificial additives or preservatives. They offer little nutritional value and can contribute to a range of health problems, from obesity to heart disease.

2. Certain Dairy Products
- For many people, especially those with specific dietary sensitivities like those on the Blood Type O diet, dairy can be problematic. It may cause inflammation, bloating, and other digestive issues. If dairy is to be included, it should be in moderation and preferably from sources known to be lower in lactose, such as goat cheese or yogurt.

3. Refined Sugars and Grains
- White bread, pasta made from white flour, and sweets should be limited. These foods can cause blood sugar spikes and crashes, leading to energy dips and increased cravings.

4. Certain Oils and Fats
- Trans fats and some saturated fats, which are often found in baked goods and fried foods, should be avoided. They contribute to bad cholesterol and can increase the risk of heart disease.

5. Alcohol and Caffeine
- While moderate consumption of alcohol and caffeine may be acceptable for some, these substances can affect digestion, sleep patterns, and overall health. They should be consumed sparingly, if at all.

Knowing which foods to embrace and which to avoid is key to optimizing your diet for health and satisfaction. Whether you're following a Blood Type Diet or another health-focused eating plan, the principle remains the same: choose whole, unprocessed foods rich in nutrients, and avoid those that your body does not handle well. This approach not only supports physical health but also enhances your mental well-being and quality of life. As always, it's wise to consult with a healthcare provider or a nutritionist to tailor your diet to your specific health needs and goals, ensuring that you get the most out of your nutritional choices.

Breakfast Recipes

1. Almond Butter Berry Shake
Servings: 2
Cooking Time: 5 minutes
Ingredients:
- 1 cup unsweetened almond milk
- 1/2 cup frozen mixed berries (blueberries, strawberries, raspberries)
- 2 tablespoons almond butter
- 1 tablespoon chia seeds
- 1/2 banana

Instructions:
1. Combine almond milk, frozen berries, almond butter, chia seeds, and banana in a blender.
2. Blend on high until smooth.
3. Pour into glasses and serve immediately.

Nutritional Info per Serving:
- Calories: 215
- Protein: 6g
- Carbohydrates: 18g
- Fat: 14g
- Fiber: 5g
- Sugar: 9g

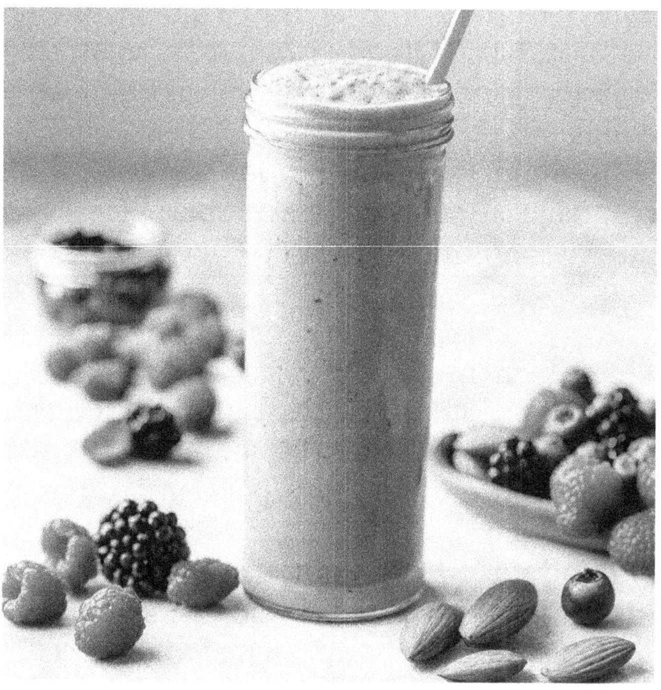

2. Pumpkin Seed Milkshake

Servings: 2
Cooking Time: 5 minutes
Ingredients:

- 1 cup unsweetened coconut milk
- 1/4 cup raw pumpkin seeds
- 1 frozen banana
- 1 tablespoon flaxseeds
- 1/2 teaspoon vanilla extract
- 1/4 teaspoon ground cinnamon

Instructions:

1. Place all ingredients in a blender.
2. Blend on high until creamy and smooth.
3. Serve chilled.

Nutritional Info per Serving:

- Calories: 238
- Protein: 7g
- Carbohydrates: 18g
- Fat: 16g
- Fiber: 4g
- Sugar: 7g

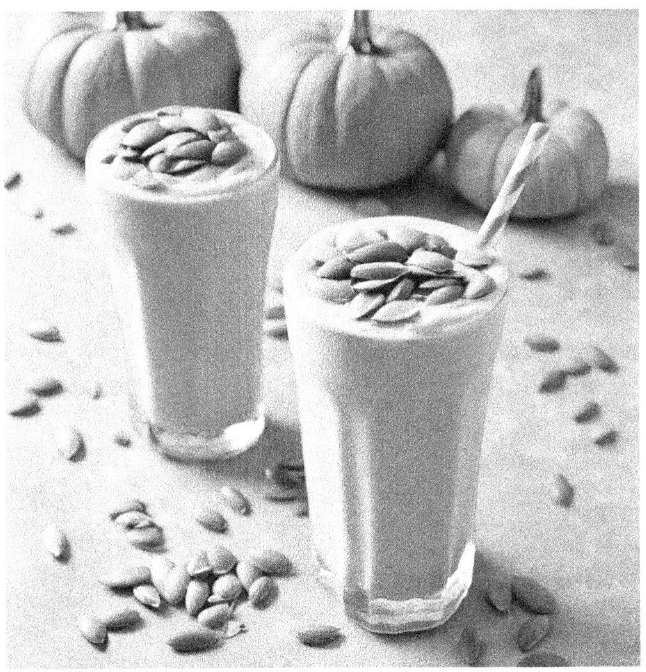

3. Beef and Spinach Breakfast Scramble

Servings: 2
Cooking Time: 15 minutes
Ingredients:

- 1/2 pound lean ground beef
- 2 cups fresh spinach, chopped
- 1 small onion, diced
- 2 cloves garlic, minced
- 1/2 teaspoon smoked paprika
- 1/4 teaspoon black pepper
- 1 tablespoon olive oil

Instructions:

1. Heat olive oil in a skillet over medium heat.
2. Add the onion and garlic, sautéing until soft.
3. Add ground beef, breaking it up as it cooks, until browned.
4. Stir in the spinach, smoked paprika, and black pepper. Cook until the spinach is wilted.
5. Serve hot.

Nutritional Info per Serving:

- Calories: 350
- Protein: 24g
- Carbohydrates: 8g
- Fat: 25g
- Fiber: 2g
- Sugar: 3g

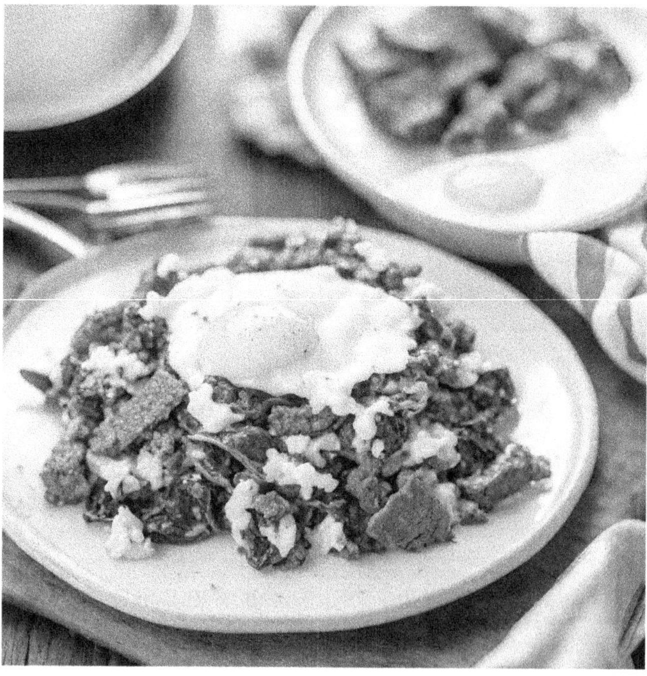

4. Turkey Bacon Avocado Cups

Servings: 2
Cooking Time: 20 minutes
Ingredients:

- 4 slices turkey bacon
- 1 ripe avocado, halved and pitted
- 2 eggs
- 1/4 teaspoon chili flakes
- Freshly ground black pepper

Instructions:

1. Preheat the oven to 400°F (200°C).
2. Line a muffin tin with turkey bacon slices, forming cups.
3. Place half an avocado in each cup, skin removed.
4. Crack an egg into each avocado half.
5. Sprinkle with chili flakes and black pepper.
6. Bake in the preheated oven for 15 minutes or until the egg whites are set.
7. Remove from the oven and serve warm.

Nutritional Info per Serving:

- Calories: 320
- Protein: 20g
- Carbohydrates: 9g
- Fat: 24g
- Fiber: 7g
- Sugar: 1g

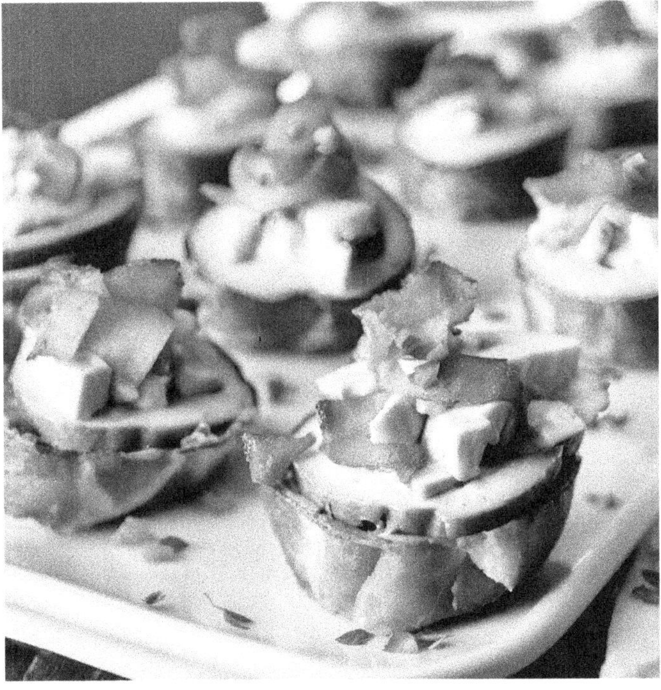

5. Smoked Salmon Omelette

Servings: 1
Cooking Time: 10 minutes
Ingredients:

- 3 eggs
- 50g smoked salmon, chopped
- 1 tablespoon chopped chives
- 1 tablespoon olive oil
- Freshly ground black pepper

Instructions:

1. Beat the eggs in a bowl and stir in the smoked salmon and chives.
2. Heat olive oil in a non-stick frying pan over medium heat.
3. Pour in the egg mixture, cooking for about 4 minutes until the edges start to lift.
4. Fold the omelette in half and continue cooking until set.
5. Season with black pepper and serve.

Nutritional Info per Serving:

- Calories: 320
- Protein: 27g
- Carbohydrates: 1g
- Fat: 23g
- Fiber: 0g
- Sugar: 1g

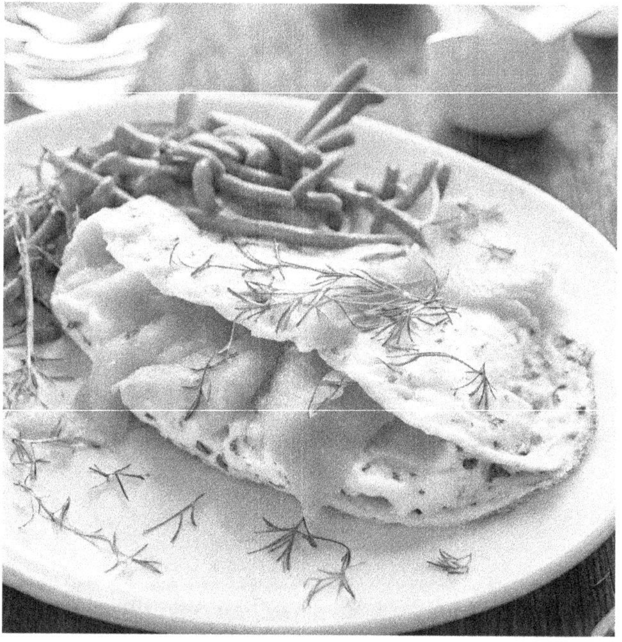

6. Buffalo Chicken Egg Muffins

Servings: 6
Cooking Time: 25 minutes
Ingredients:

- 6 eggs
- 1/2 cup cooked chicken breast, shredded
- 1/4 cup hot sauce
- 1/4 cup chopped celery
- 1 tablespoon olive oil
- Chili flakes

Instructions:

1. Preheat the oven to 375°F (190°C).
2. In a bowl, combine eggs, chicken, hot sauce, and celery.
3. Grease a muffin tin with olive oil.
4. Pour the mixture into the muffin cups.
5. Sprinkle chili flakes on top.
6. Bake for 20 minutes, or until the muffins are set.
7. Serve warm.

Nutritional Info per Muffin:

- Calories: 120
- Protein: 10g
- Carbohydrates: 1g
- Fat: 8g
- Fiber: 0g
- Sugar: 0g

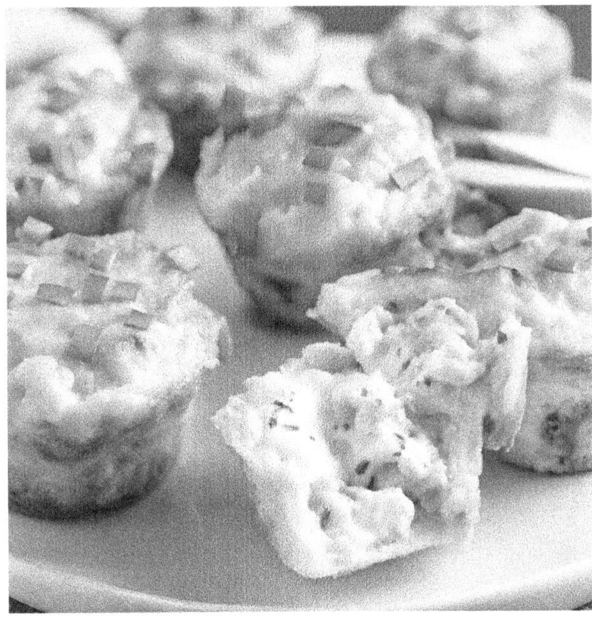

7. Sardine and Cucumber Salad

Servings: 2

Cooking Time: 5 minutes

Ingredients:

- 1 can sardines in olive oil, drained
- 1 cucumber, sliced
- 1 tablespoon lemon juice
- 1 tablespoon chopped fresh dill
- Freshly ground black pepper

Instructions:

1. In a bowl, combine sardines and cucumber slices.
2. Drizzle with lemon juice and sprinkle with dill.
3. Toss gently to mix.
4. Season with black pepper and serve chilled.

Nutritional Info per Serving:

- Calories: 180
- Protein: 12g
- Carbohydrates: 4g
- Fat: 13g
- Fiber: 1g
- Sugar: 2g

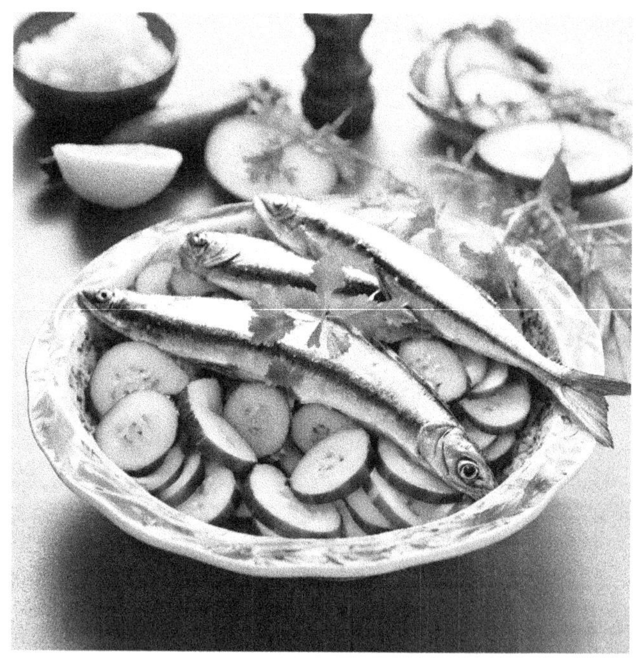

8. Lamb Breakfast Patties

Servings: 4
Cooking Time: 15 minutes
Ingredients:

- 1 pound ground lamb
- 1 teaspoon cumin
- 1 teaspoon smoked paprika
- 1 clove garlic, minced
- 1 tablespoon olive oil
- Chili flakes

Instructions:

1. In a bowl, mix ground lamb with cumin, smoked paprika, garlic, and chili flakes.
2. Form into 8 small patties.
3. Heat olive oil in a skillet over medium heat.
4. Cook patties for about 5-7 minutes on each side until fully cooked.
5. Serve hot.

Nutritional Info per Serving:

- Calories: 300
- Protein: 19g
- Carbohydrates: 1g
- Fat: 24g
- Fiber: 0g
- Sugar: 0g

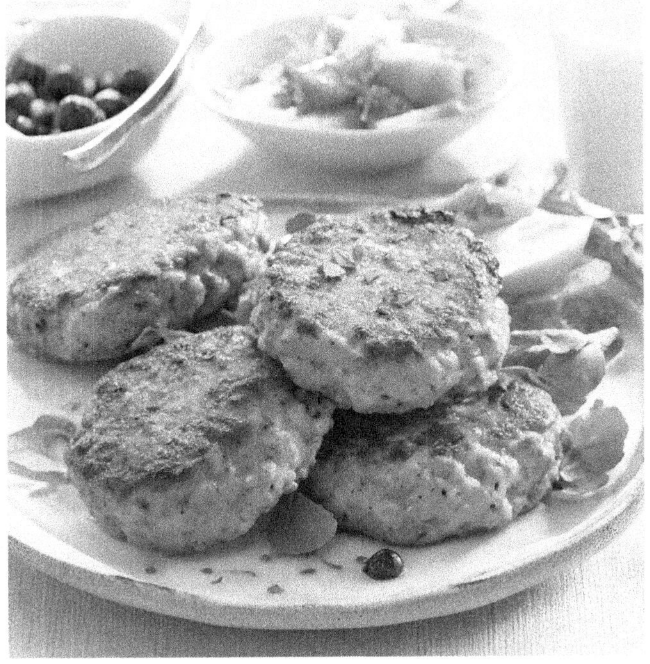

9. Venison and Vegetable Stir-Fry

Servings: 2

Cooking Time: 20 minutes

Ingredients:

- 1/2 pound venison, thinly sliced
- 1 bell pepper, sliced
- 1/2 onion, sliced
- 2 tablespoons coconut oil
- 1 tablespoon soy sauce
- 1 teaspoon sesame seeds
- Freshly ground black pepper

Instructions:

1. Heat coconut oil in a wok or large skillet over high heat.
2. Add venison slices and stir-fry for 5 minutes.
3. Add bell pepper and onion, continuing to stir-fry until vegetables are tender and venison is cooked through.
4. Stir in soy sauce and sprinkle with sesame seeds.
5. Season with black pepper and serve hot.

Nutritional Info per Serving:

- Calories: 350
- Protein: 24g
- Carbohydrates: 9g
- Fat: 24g
- Fiber: 2g
- Sugar: 5g

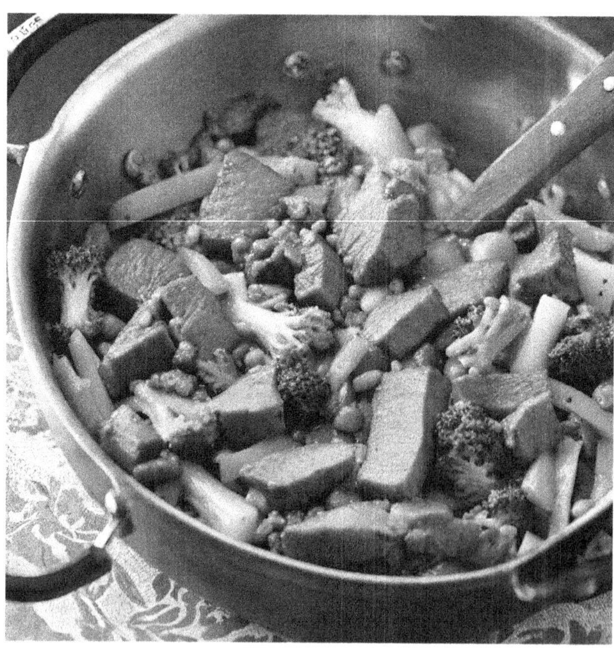

10. Egg, Kale, and Beef Stir Fry

Servings: 2

Cooking Time: 15 minutes

Ingredients:

- 4 eggs, beaten
- 1/2 pound ground beef
- 2 cups kale, chopped
- 1 tablespoon olive oil
- 1 teaspoon garlic powder
- Freshly ground black pepper

Instructions:

1. Heat olive oil in a skillet over medium heat.
2. Add ground beef and cook until browned.
3. Stir in kale and cook until wilted.
4. Pour eggs over the beef and kale mixture, stirring until the eggs are fully cooked.
5. Season with garlic powder and black pepper.
6. Serve hot.

Nutritional Info per Serving:

- Calories: 400
- Protein: 28g
- Carbohydrates: 5g
- Fat: 30g
- Fiber: 1g
- Sugar: 1g

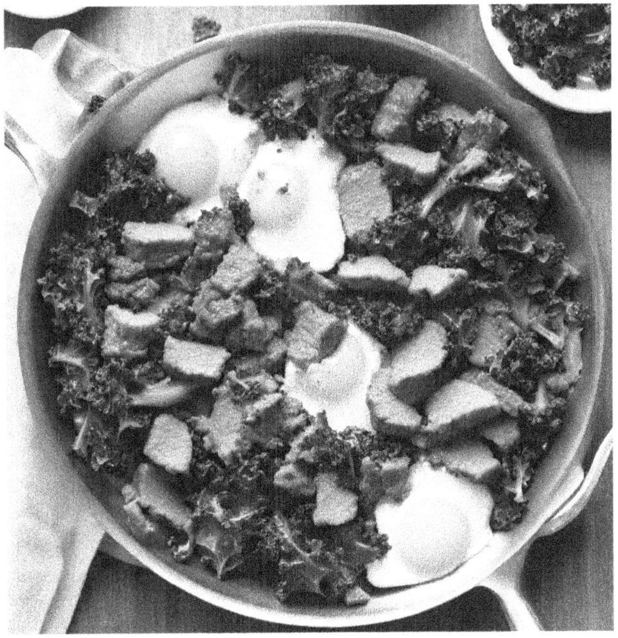

11. Mackerel and Tomato Salad

Servings: 2
Cooking Time: 10 minutes
Ingredients:

- 2 mackerel fillets, grilled and flaked
- 2 tomatoes, chopped
- 1/4 red onion, finely sliced
- 1 tablespoon olive oil
- 1 tablespoon lemon juice
- Freshly ground black pepper

Instructions:

1. In a bowl, combine mackerel, tomatoes, and red onion.
2. Drizzle with olive oil and lemon juice.
3. Toss to combine.
4. Season with black pepper and serve chilled.

Nutritional Info per Serving:

- Calories: 290
- Protein: 22g
- Carbohydrates: 6g
- Fat: 20g
- Fiber: 2g
- Sugar: 4g

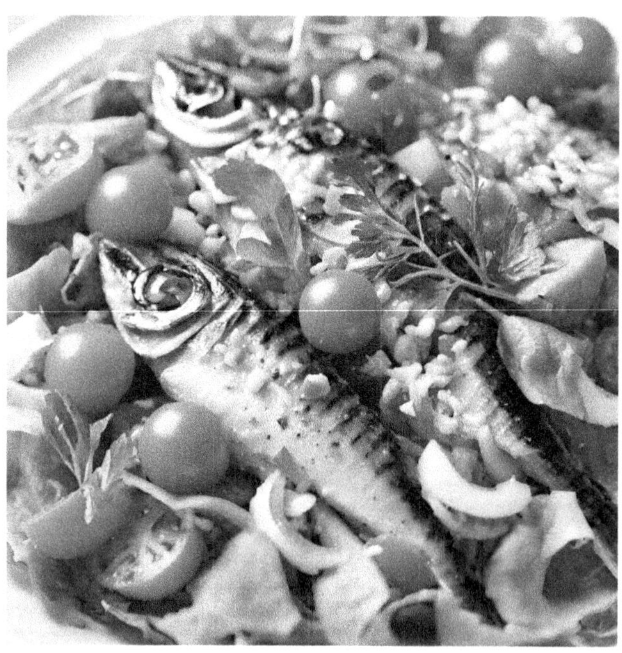

12. Berry Salad with Lemon Dressing

Servings: 2

Cooking Time: 10 minutes

Ingredients:

- 1 cup fresh strawberries, halved
- 1 cup fresh blueberries
- 1 cup fresh raspberries
- 1 tablespoon fresh lemon juice
- 2 teaspoons honey
- 1 tablespoon olive oil
- Fresh mint leaves for garnish

Instructions:

1. In a large bowl, combine strawberries, blueberries, and raspberries.
2. In a small bowl, whisk together lemon juice, honey, and olive oil until well combined.
3. Pour dressing over the berries and gently toss.
4. Garnish with mint leaves and serve immediately.

Nutritional Info per Serving:

- Calories: 180
- Protein: 2g
- Carbohydrates: 34g
- Fat: 6g
- Fiber: 8g
- Sugar: 20g

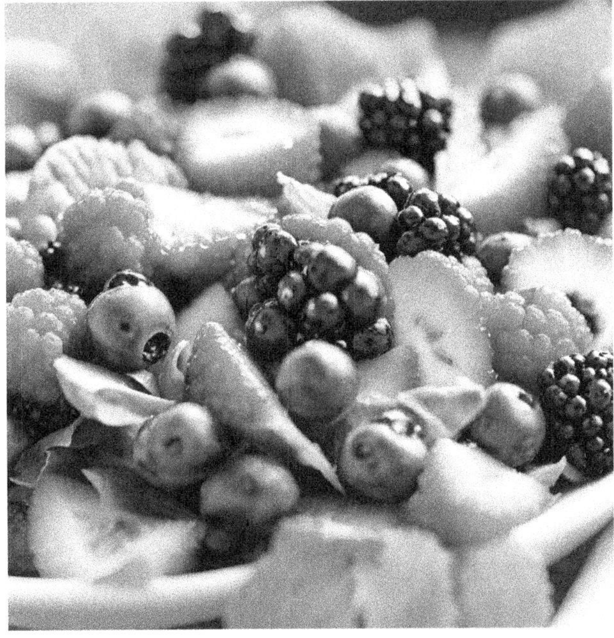

13. Green Smoothie Bowl

Servings: 1

Cooking Time: 5 minutes

Ingredients:

- 1 cup fresh spinach
- 1/2 ripe avocado
- 1/2 banana
- 1/2 cup coconut water
- 1 tablespoon chia seeds
- 1/4 cup sliced almonds for topping

Instructions:

1. In a blender, combine spinach, avocado, banana, and coconut water. Blend until smooth.
2. Pour the smoothie into a bowl.
3. Top with chia seeds and sliced almonds.
4. Serve immediately.

Nutritional Info per Serving:

- Calories: 350
- Protein: 7g
- Carbohydrates: 31g
- Fat: 24g
- Fiber: 10g
- Sugar: 12g

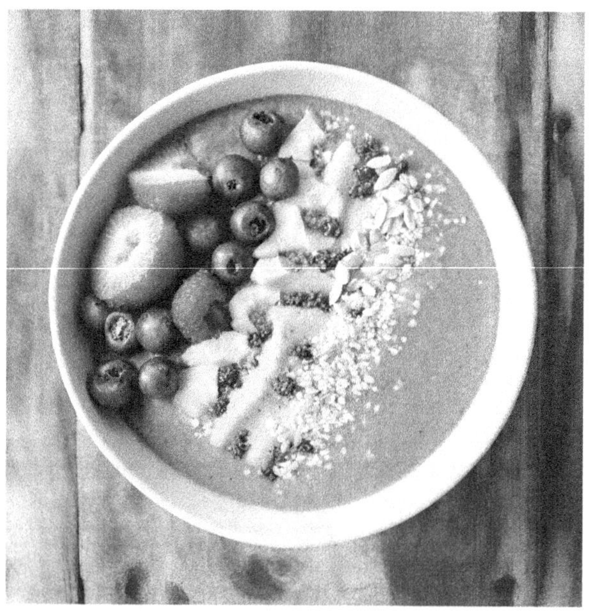

14. Avocado Smoothie

Servings: 1
Cooking Time: 5 minutes
Ingredients:

- 1 ripe avocado
- 1 cup unsweetened almond milk
- 1 tablespoon lime juice
- 1 tablespoon honey

Instructions:

1. Combine all ingredients in a blender.
2. Blend until smooth and creamy.
3. Serve chilled.

Nutritional Info per Serving:

- Calories: 340
- Protein: 4g
- Carbohydrates: 24g
- Fat: 26g
- Fiber: 10g
- Sugar: 12g

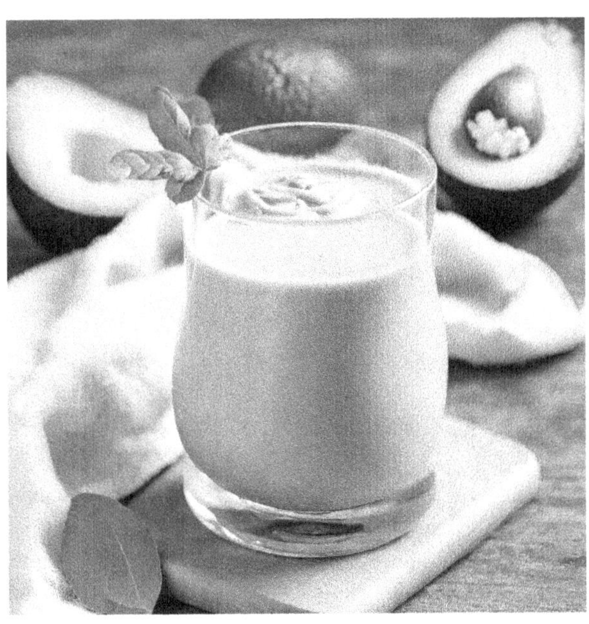

15. Melon Medley with Mint

Servings: 2
Cooking Time: 10 minutes
Ingredients:

- 1 cup cantaloupe, cubed
- 1 cup honeydew melon, cubed
- 1/2 cup watermelon, cubed
- 1 tablespoon fresh mint, chopped
- 1 tablespoon lime juice

Instructions:

1. In a large bowl, combine all melon cubes.
2. Sprinkle with chopped mint.
3. Drizzle lime juice over the top and gently toss to combine.
4. Serve chilled.

Nutritional Info per Serving:

- Calories: 60
- Protein: 1g
- Carbohydrates: 15g
- Fat: 0g
- Fiber: 1g
- Sugar: 13g

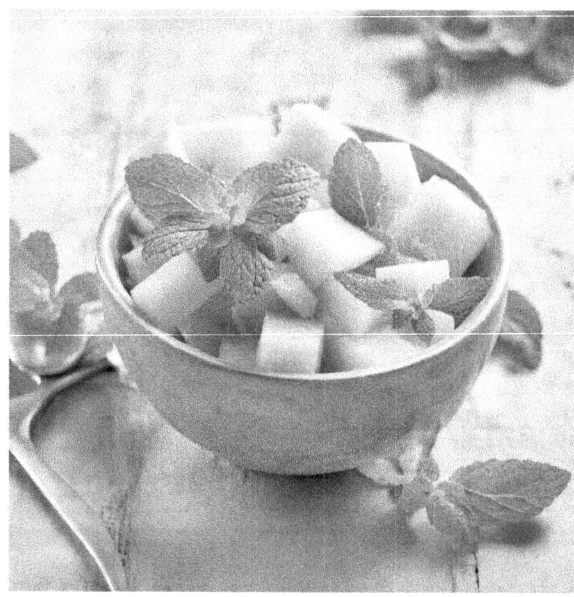

16. Citrusy Shrimp Salad

Servings: 2
Cooking Time: 15 minutes
Ingredients:
- 200g cooked shrimp, peeled
- 1 orange, peeled and segmented
- 1 grapefruit, peeled and segmented
- 1 avocado, sliced
- 1 tablespoon olive oil
- 1 tablespoon lemon juice
- Fresh cilantro for garnish

Instructions:
1. In a salad bowl, combine shrimp, orange segments, grapefruit segments, and avocado slices.
2. Drizzle with olive oil and lemon juice.
3. Garnish with fresh cilantro.
4. Serve immediately.

Nutritional Info per Serving:
- Calories: 290
- Protein: 18g
- Carbohydrates: 20g
- Fat: 17g
- Fiber: 6g
- Sugar: 12g

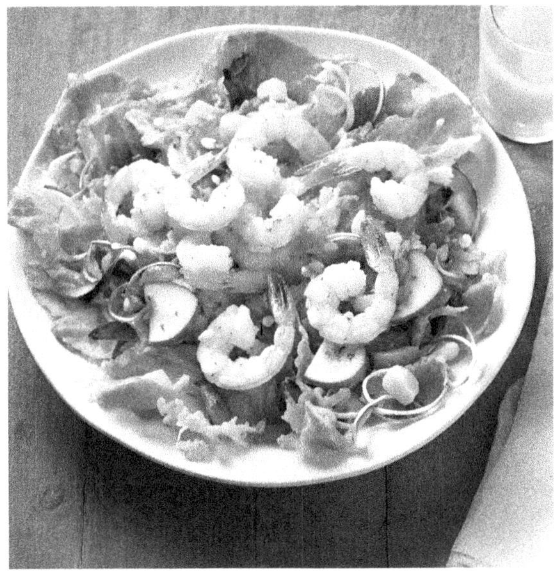

17. Chilled Berry Soup

Servings: 2
Cooking Time: 10 minutes (plus chilling time)
Ingredients:

- 1 cup strawberries, hulled
- 1 cup raspberries
- 1/2 cup blueberries
- 1 cup unsweetened apple juice
- 1/2 cup coconut cream
- 1 tablespoon honey
- Fresh mint leaves for garnish

Instructions:

1. In a blender, combine all berries and apple juice. Blend until smooth.
2. Pass the mixture through a sieve to remove seeds.
3. Stir in coconut cream and honey.
4. Chill in the refrigerator for at least 1 hour.
5. Serve cold, garnished with mint leaves.

Nutritional Info per Serving:

- Calories: 210
- Protein: 2g
- Carbohydrates: 37g
- Fat: 7g
- Fiber: 7g
- Sugar: 28g

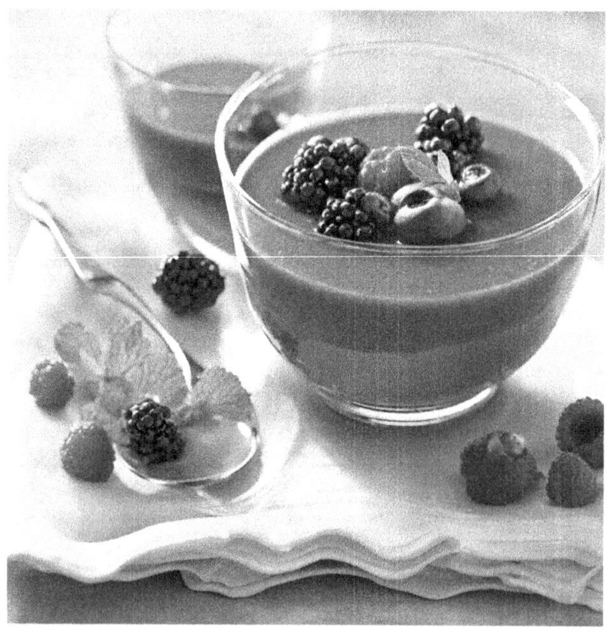

18. Chicken Liver Pâté with Cucumber Slices

Servings: 4
Cooking Time: 30 minutes
Ingredients:

- 1 pound chicken livers, cleaned
- 1/4 cup butter
- 1 onion, finely chopped
- 1 clove garlic, minced
- 1/4 cup brandy
- 1 teaspoon thyme leaves
- Freshly ground black pepper
- Cucumber slices for serving

Instructions:

1. Melt half the butter in a skillet over medium heat.
2. Add onion and garlic, sautéing until soft.
3. Increase heat, add chicken livers and cook until browned on all sides.
4. Pour in brandy, allowing it to evaporate.
5. Transfer to a food processor, add thyme and remaining butter, and blend until smooth.
6. Season with black pepper.
7. Refrigerate until firm, about 2 hours.
8. Serve with cucumber slices.

Nutritional Info per Serving:

- Calories: 292
- Protein: 19g
- Carbohydrates: 5g
- Fat: 21g
- Fiber: 0g
- Sugar: 2g

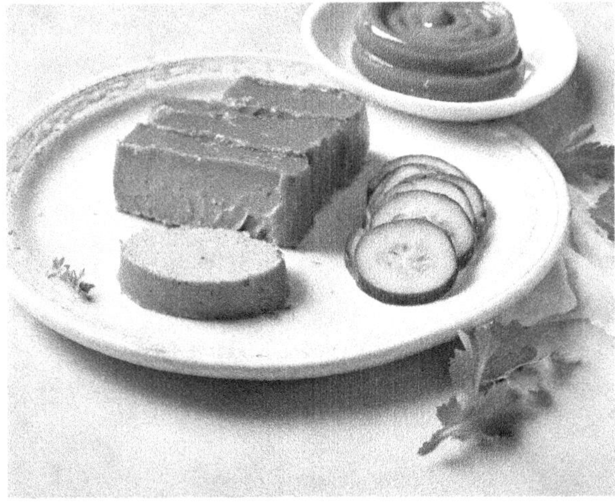

19. Herbed Turkey Patties

Servings: 4
Cooking Time: 20 minutes
Ingredients:

- 1 pound ground turkey
- 1 tablespoon chopped fresh parsley
- 1 tablespoon chopped fresh basil
- 1 teaspoon dried oregano
- 1 clove garlic, minced
- 1 tablespoon olive oil
- Freshly ground black pepper

Instructions:

1. In a bowl, combine ground turkey, parsley, basil, oregano, and garlic.
2. Form the mixture into 8 small patties.
3. Heat olive oil in a skillet over medium heat.
4. Cook the patties for about 4-5 minutes on each side until golden and cooked through.
5. Season with black pepper and serve.

Nutritional Info per Serving:

- Calories: 180
- Protein: 22g
- Carbohydrates: 1g
- Fat: 10g
- Fiber: 0g
- Sugar: 0g

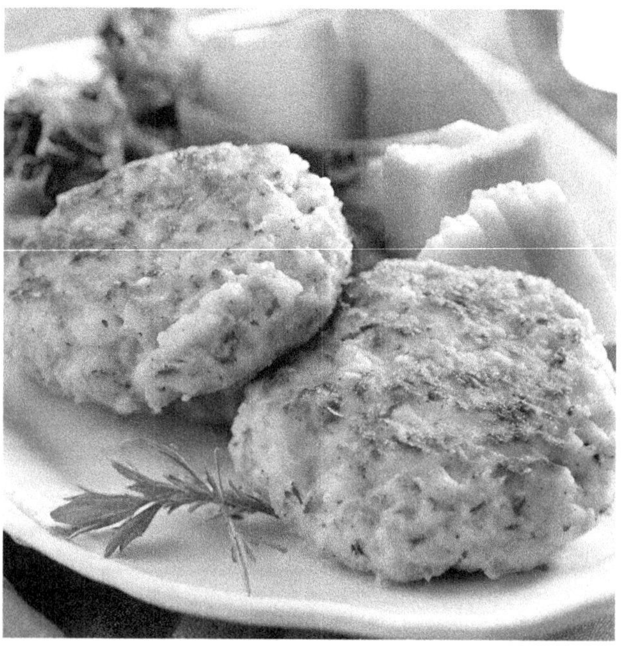

20. Beef Tartare

Servings: 2

Cooking Time: 15 minutes (preparation only)

Ingredients:

- 1/2 pound high-quality raw beef fillet, finely chopped
- 1 small shallot, minced
- 1 teaspoon capers, chopped
- 1 tablespoon olive oil
- 1 teaspoon Dijon mustard
- 1 raw egg yolk
- Freshly ground black pepper
- Fresh parsley, chopped for garnish

Instructions:

1. In a mixing bowl, combine the chopped beef, shallot, capers, olive oil, and Dijon mustard.
2. Carefully place an egg yolk on top of each portion.
3. Season with black pepper.
4. Garnish with chopped parsley.
5. Serve immediately with whole-grain toast if desired.

Nutritional Info per Serving:

- Calories: 300
- Protein: 24g
- Carbohydrates: 2g
- Fat: 22g
- Fiber: 0g
- Sugar: 1g

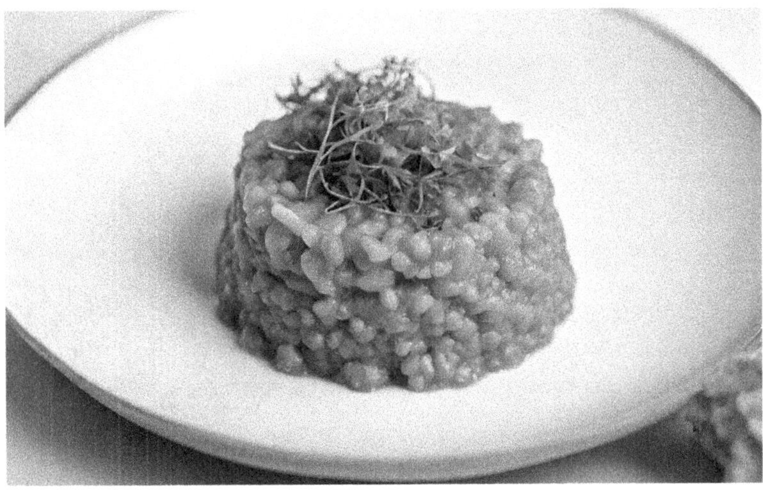

21. Salmon and Avocado Towers
Servings: 2
Cooking Time: 10 minutes
Ingredients:

- 200g smoked salmon
- 1 ripe avocado, diced
- 1 tablespoon lemon juice
- 1/4 red onion, finely chopped
- 1 tablespoon capers
- Freshly ground black pepper

Instructions:

1. In a bowl, gently mix the diced avocado with lemon juice and red onion.
2. Use a round mold or a cup to layer the avocado mixture and smoked salmon alternately in a tower shape on the plate.
3. Top with capers.
4. Season with black pepper.
5. Carefully remove the mold and serve.

Nutritional Info per Serving:

- Calories: 290
- Protein: 21g
- Carbohydrates: 9g
- Fat: 20g
- Fiber: 4g
- Sugar: 2g

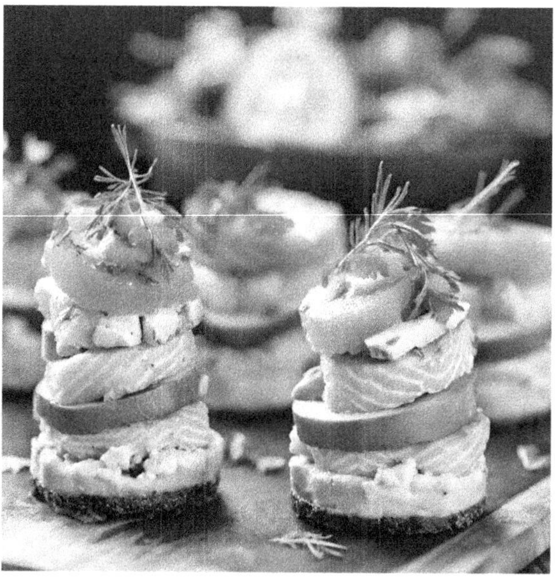

22. Chicken and Spinach Crepes

Servings: 4

Cooking Time: 30 minutes

Ingredients:

- For the crepes:
    - 1 cup all-purpose flour (or a suitable gluten-free alternative)
    - 2 eggs
    - 1/2 cup water
    - 1/2 cup milk
    - 2 tablespoons melted butter
- For the filling:
    - 1/2 pound cooked chicken breast, shredded
    - 2 cups fresh spinach, wilted
    - 1/4 cup cream cheese
    - 1 teaspoon nutmeg
    - Freshly ground black pepper

Instructions:

1. Prepare crepes: In a blender, mix flour, eggs, water, milk, and butter until smooth. Let the batter sit for a few minutes.
2. Heat a non-stick skillet over medium heat. Pour a small amount of batter into the pan, swirling to spread evenly. Cook for about 2 minutes per side. Repeat with remaining batter.
3. Prepare filling: In a bowl, mix shredded chicken, wilted spinach, cream cheese, and nutmeg.
4. Assemble crepes: Spoon filling onto each crepe, fold, and serve.
5. Season with black pepper.

Nutritional Info per Serving:

- Calories: 330
- Protein: 28g
- Carbohydrates: 23g
- Fat: 15g
- Fiber: 2g
- Sugar: 3g

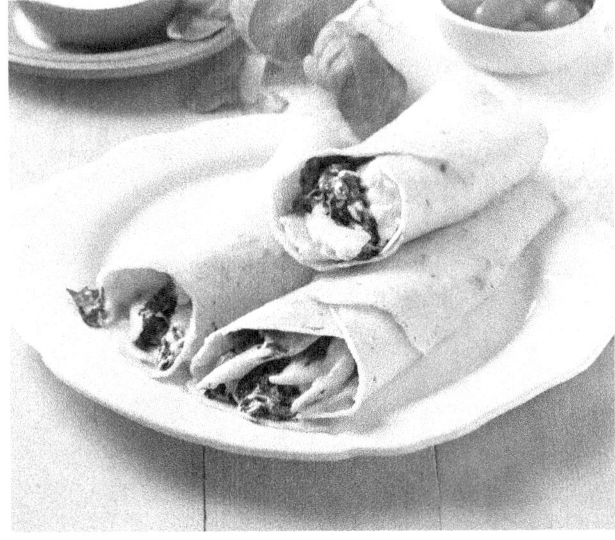

Poultry Recipes

1. Chicken Zucchini Boats
Servings: 4
Cooking Time: 30 minutes
Ingredients:
- 4 medium zucchinis, halved lengthwise
- 1 pound ground chicken
- 1 small onion, finely chopped
- 1 bell pepper, finely chopped
- 2 cloves garlic, minced
- 1 cup tomato sauce
- 1 tablespoon olive oil
- Freshly ground black pepper
- Fresh basil for garnish

Instructions:
1. Preheat the oven to 375°F (190°C).
2. Scoop out the center of each zucchini half to create a "boat."
3. In a skillet, heat olive oil over medium heat. Add onion, bell pepper, and garlic; sauté until soft.
4. Add ground chicken and cook until browned.
5. Stir in tomato sauce and cook for an additional 5 minutes.
6. Fill zucchini boats with the chicken mixture.
7. Place filled zucchinis on a baking sheet and bake for 20 minutes.
8. Garnish with fresh basil and black pepper before serving.

Nutritional Info per Serving:
- Calories: 265
- Protein: 26g
- Carbohydrates: 15g
- Fat: 12g
- Fiber: 3g
- Sugar: 8g

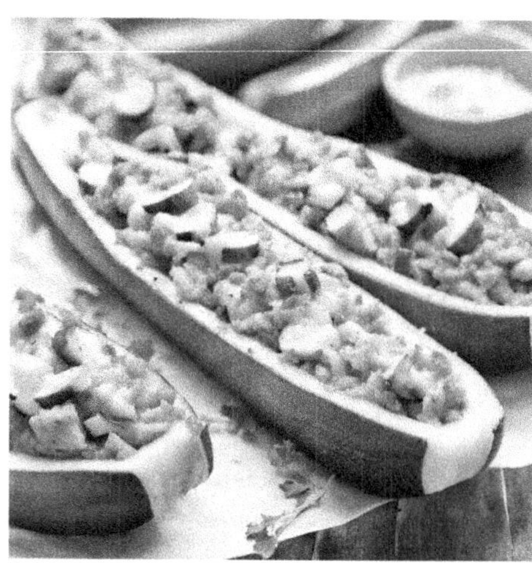

2. Peppered Chicken Liver

Servings: 4

Cooking Time: 15 minutes

Ingredients:

- 1 pound chicken livers, cleaned and trimmed
- 2 tablespoons olive oil
- 1 teaspoon cracked black pepper
- 1/2 teaspoon smoked paprika
- Juice of 1 lemon
- Fresh parsley, chopped for garnish

Instructions:

1. Heat olive oil in a skillet over medium-high heat.
2. Add chicken livers and sauté until browned on all sides, about 5 minutes.
3. Sprinkle with black pepper and smoked paprika during cooking.
4. Just before removing from heat, pour lemon juice over the livers.
5. Garnish with fresh parsley and serve immediately.

Nutritional Info per Serving:

- Calories: 210
- Protein: 19g
- Carbohydrates: 1g
- Fat: 14g
- Fiber: 0g
- Sugar: 0g

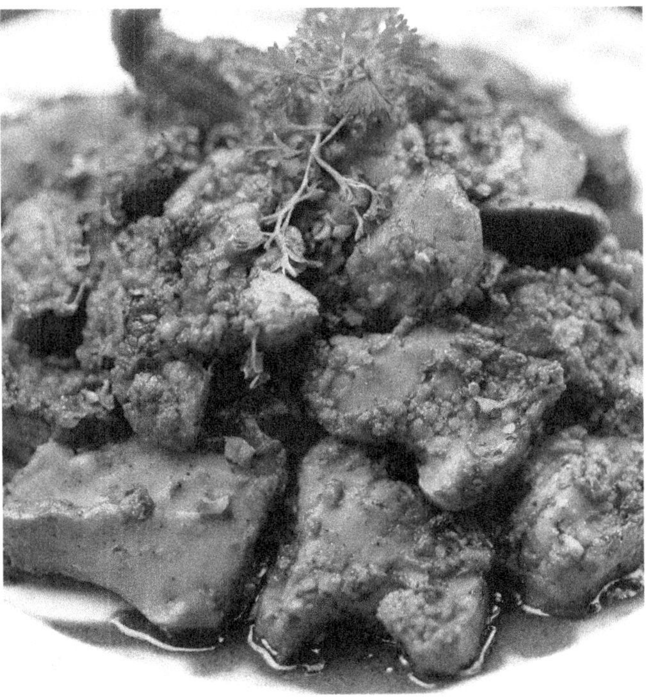

3. Garlic and Herb Roasted Chicken Thighs

Servings: 4
Cooking Time: 45 minutes
Ingredients:

- 8 chicken thighs, bone-in and skin-on
- 4 cloves garlic, minced
- 1 tablespoon fresh rosemary, chopped
- 1 tablespoon fresh thyme, chopped
- 2 tablespoons olive oil
- Freshly ground black pepper
- Lemon wedges for serving

Instructions:

1. Preheat oven to 400°F (200°C).
2. In a small bowl, mix garlic, rosemary, thyme, and olive oil.
3. Rub the herb mixture all over the chicken thighs.
4. Arrange chicken in a single layer in a baking dish.
5. Roast in the oven for 35-40 minutes, or until the skin is crispy and the chicken is cooked through.
6. Serve with lemon wedges and season with black pepper.

Nutritional Info per Serving:

- Calories: 400
- Protein: 31g
- Carbohydrates: 2g
- Fat: 29g
- Fiber: 0g
- Sugar: 0g

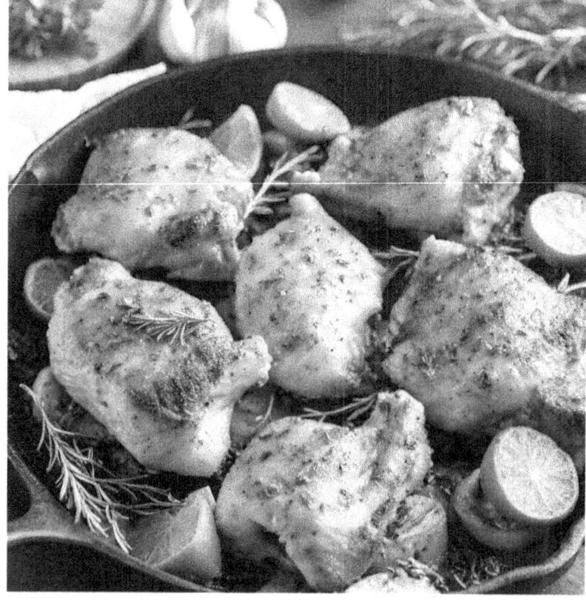

4. Grilled Quail with Lemon Herb Marinade

Servings: 4

Cooking Time: 25 minutes (plus marinating time)

Ingredients:

- 4 quail, cleaned and split
- 1/4 cup olive oil
- Juice of 1 lemon
- 1 tablespoon fresh rosemary, chopped
- 1 tablespoon fresh thyme, chopped
- Freshly ground black pepper
- Lemon slices for garnish

Instructions:

1. In a bowl, combine olive oil, lemon juice, rosemary, and thyme.
2. Marinate the quail in this mixture for at least 2 hours in the refrigerator.
3. Preheat grill to medium-high heat.
4. Remove quail from marinade, season with black pepper, and grill for about 10 minutes on each side or until cooked through.
5. Serve with lemon slices.

Nutritional Info per Serving:

- Calories: 290
- Protein: 24g
- Carbohydrates: 1g
- Fat: 21g
- Fiber: 0g
- Sugar: 0g

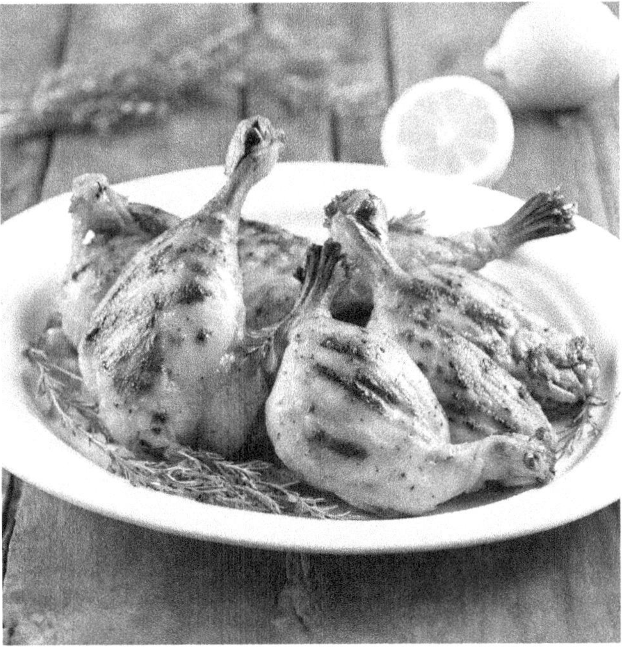

5. Duck Fat Sautéed Greens

Servings: 4

Cooking Time: 15 minutes

Ingredients:

- 4 cups mixed greens (such as kale and spinach)
- 3 tablespoons duck fat
- 2 cloves garlic, minced
- Freshly ground black pepper
- Lemon wedges for serving

Instructions:

1. Heat duck fat in a large skillet over medium heat.
2. Add garlic and sauté for about 1 minute until fragrant.
3. Add the greens and cook, stirring frequently, until wilted and tender, about 5-7 minutes.
4. Season with black pepper.
5. Serve hot with lemon wedges on the side.

Nutritional Info per Serving:

- Calories: 150
- Protein: 2g
- Carbohydrates: 4g
- Fat: 14g
- Fiber: 2g
- Sugar: 1g

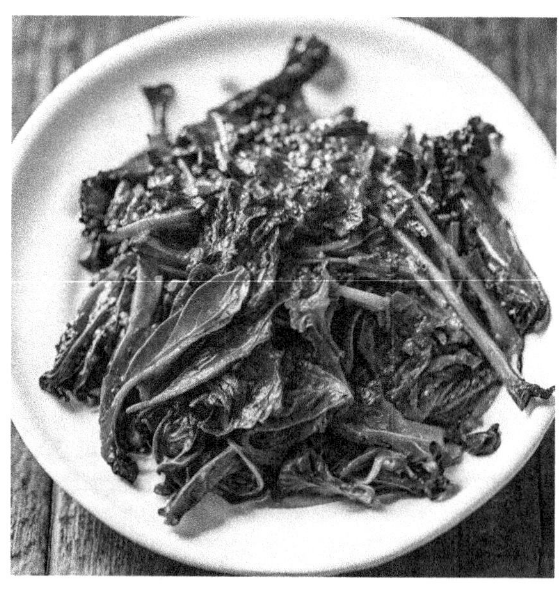

6. Pan-Seared Pheasant with Vegetables

Servings: 4

Cooking Time: 30 minutes

Ingredients:

- 2 pheasants, quartered
- 2 tablespoons olive oil
- 1 cup carrots, sliced
- 1 cup celery, sliced
- 1 onion, sliced
- Freshly ground black pepper
- Fresh herbs (such as thyme and rosemary) for garnish

Instructions:

1. Heat olive oil in a large skillet over medium-high heat.
2. Add pheasant pieces and sear on all sides until golden brown, about 5 minutes per side.
3. Reduce heat to medium, add carrots, celery, and onion to the skillet, and cook until the vegetables are tender and the pheasant is cooked through, about 15-20 minutes.
4. Season with black pepper and garnish with fresh herbs.
5. Serve hot.

Nutritional Info per Serving:

- Calories: 310
- Protein: 35g
- Carbohydrates: 9g
- Fat: 15g
- Fiber: 2g
- Sugar: 4g

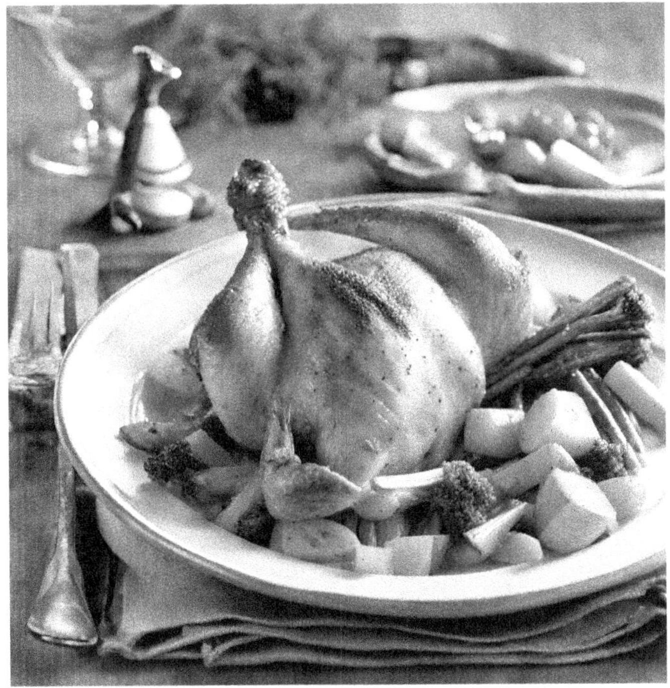

7. Herb-Stuffed Game Hen

Servings: 4
Cooking Time: 1 hour
Ingredients:

- 2 game hens, halved
- 1/4 cup fresh parsley, chopped
- 1 tablespoon fresh thyme, chopped
- 1 tablespoon fresh rosemary, chopped
- 2 cloves garlic, minced
- 2 tablespoons olive oil
- Freshly ground black pepper

Instructions:

1. Preheat oven to 375°F (190°C).
2. In a small bowl, mix together parsley, thyme, rosemary, and garlic.
3. Stuff each game hen half with the herb mixture.
4. Rub the outside of each hen with olive oil and season with black pepper.
5. Roast in the preheated oven for about 45-50 minutes, or until the hens are golden brown and cooked through.
6. Serve hot.

Nutritional Info per Serving:

- Calories: 400
- Protein: 30g
- Carbohydrates: 2g
- Fat: 30g
- Fiber: 1g
- Sugar: 0g

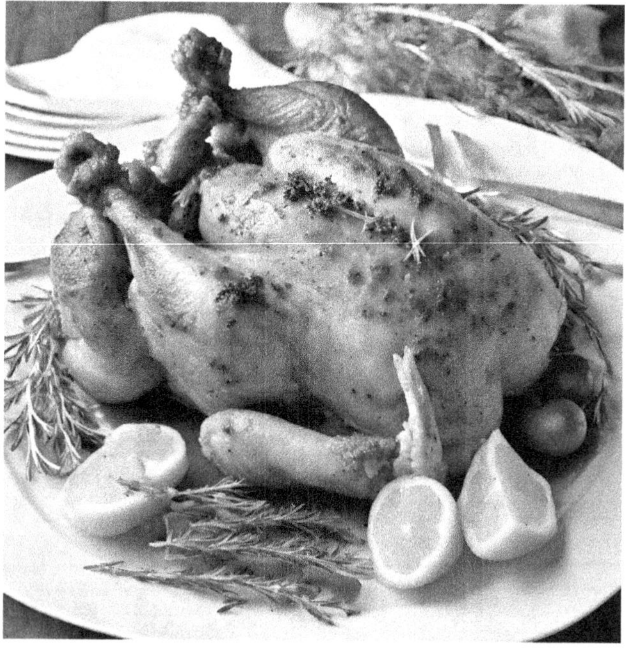

8. Spiced Duck Legs

Servings: 4

Cooking Time: 1 hour 20 minutes

Ingredients:

- 4 duck legs
- 1 tablespoon paprika
- 1 teaspoon ground cumin
- 1 teaspoon ground coriander
- 1/2 teaspoon ground cinnamon
- 2 tablespoons olive oil
- Freshly ground black pepper

Instructions:

1. Preheat oven to 350°F (175°C).
2. In a small bowl, combine paprika, cumin, coriander, and cinnamon.
3. Rub the spice mix all over the duck legs.
4. Heat olive oil in a large oven-proof skillet over medium heat. Add duck legs and sear until browned on all sides.
5. Transfer the skillet to the oven and roast for about 1 hour, or until the duck is tender and the skin is crisp.
6. Season with black pepper.
7. Serve hot.

Nutritional Info per Serving:

- Calories: 510
- Protein: 30g
- Carbohydrates: 2g
- Fat: 44g
- Fiber: 1g
- Sugar: 0g

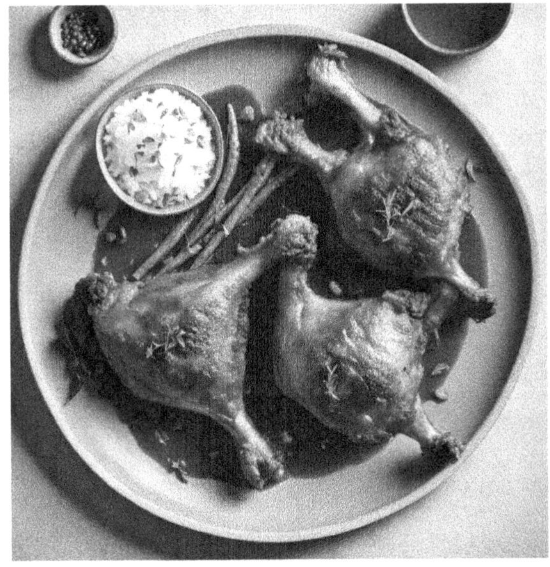

9. Barbecue Quail

Servings: 4

Cooking Time: 30 minutes

Ingredients:

- 4 quails, cleaned and split
- 1/2 cup barbecue sauce (choose a gluten-free, low-sugar variety)
- 2 tablespoons olive oil
- Freshly ground black pepper
- Fresh herbs (such as parsley or thyme) for garnish

Instructions:

1. Preheat your grill to medium-high heat.
2. Brush each quail with olive oil and season with black pepper.
3. Grill the quail for about 5 minutes on each side or until nicely charred and nearly cooked through.
4. Brush the barbecue sauce over the quail and grill for an additional 5 minutes to caramelize the sauce.
5. Garnish with fresh herbs before serving.

Nutritional Info per Serving:

- Calories: 280
- Protein: 24g
- Carbohydrates: 8g
- Fat: 18g
- Fiber: 1g
- Sugar: 6g

10. Pheasant in Herb Butter

Servings: 4
Cooking Time: 1 hour
Ingredients:

- 2 pheasants, cleaned and quartered
- 1/4 cup butter, softened
- 1 tablespoon fresh thyme, minced
- 1 tablespoon fresh parsley, minced
- 1 clove garlic, minced
- Freshly ground black pepper

Instructions:

1. Preheat oven to 375°F (190°C).
2. In a small bowl, combine the butter, thyme, parsley, and garlic.
3. Rub the herb butter mixture all over the pheasant pieces.
4. Place the pheasant in a roasting pan and season with black pepper.
5. Roast in the preheated oven for about 50 minutes or until the pheasant is golden and cooked through.
6. Serve hot, garnished with additional herbs if desired.

Nutritional Info per Serving:

- Calories: 360
- Protein: 34g
- Carbohydrates: 1g
- Fat: 24g
- Fiber: 0g
- Sugar: 0g

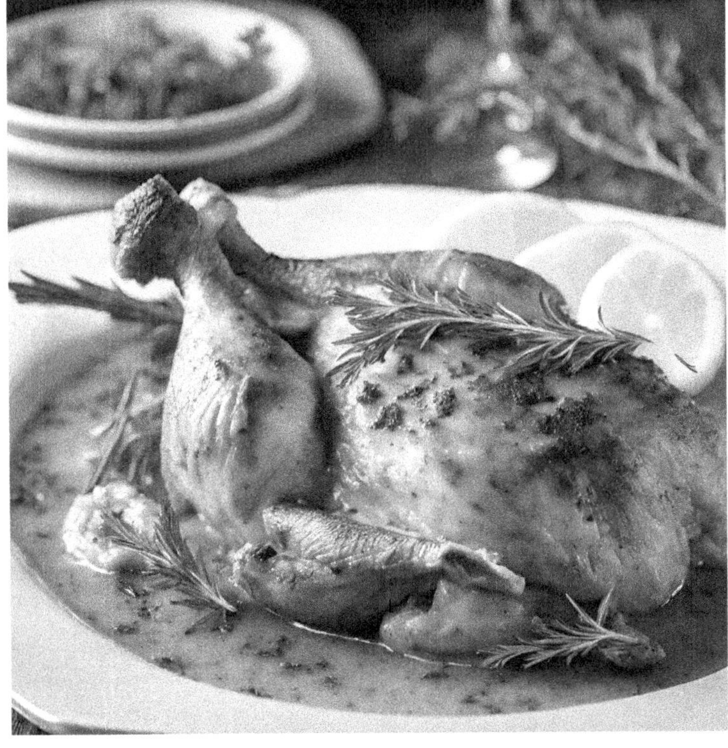

11. Duck Breast with Cherry Sauce

Servings: 4

Cooking Time: 40 minutes

Ingredients:

- 4 duck breasts, skin scored
- 1 cup fresh or frozen cherries, pitted
- 1/4 cup red wine
- 1 tablespoon balsamic vinegar
- 1 teaspoon honey
- Freshly ground black pepper

Instructions:

1. Preheat your oven to 400°F (200°C).
2. Place duck breasts skin-side down in a cold non-stick skillet.
3. Turn heat to medium and cook until the skin is crispy, about 6-7 minutes.
4. Flip the duck, then transfer the skillet to the oven and roast for 6-8 minutes for medium-rare.
5. Meanwhile, in a saucepan, combine cherries, red wine, balsamic vinegar, and honey. Simmer over medium heat until the sauce thickens, about 10 minutes.
6. Season the sauce with black pepper.
7. Slice the duck and serve with the cherry sauce.

Nutritional Info per Serving:

- Calories: 420
- Protein: 30g
- Carbohydrates: 11g
- Fat: 28g
- Fiber: 1g
- Sugar: 9g

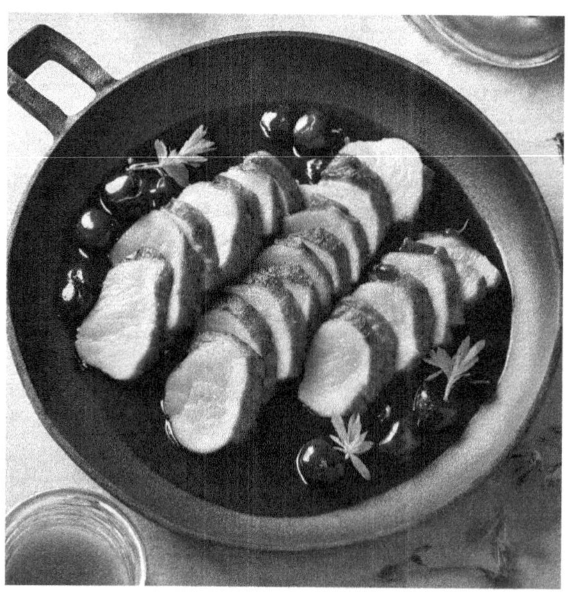

12. Grilled Game Hen

Servings: 4

Cooking Time: 50 minutes

Ingredients:

- 2 game hens, split in half
- 2 tablespoons olive oil
- 1 tablespoon fresh rosemary, minced
- 1 tablespoon fresh thyme, minced
- Freshly ground black pepper
- Lemon wedges for serving

Instructions:

1. Preheat your grill to medium-high heat.
2. Rub each hen half with olive oil and the minced herbs.
3. Season with black pepper.
4. Grill the hens, turning occasionally, until the skin is crisp and the meat is cooked through, about 40-45 minutes.
5. Serve with lemon wedges.

Nutritional Info per Serving:

- Calories: 310
- Protein: 28g
- Carbohydrates: 0g
- Fat: 22g
- Fiber: 0g
- Sugar: 0g

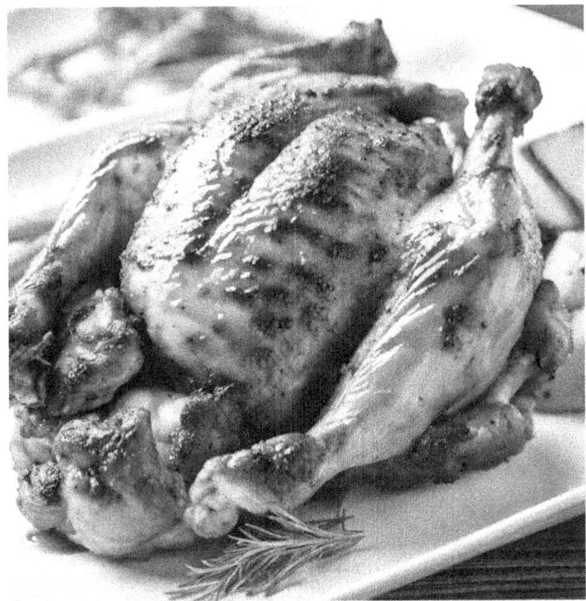

13. Chicken Liver Pâté

Servings: 4
Cooking Time: 30 minutes
Ingredients:

- 1 pound chicken livers, cleaned
- 1/4 cup butter
- 1 onion, finely chopped
- 1 clove garlic, minced
- 1/4 cup cream
- Freshly ground black pepper
- Fresh thyme for garnish

Instructions:

1. In a skillet, melt half the butter over medium heat. Add onion and garlic and sauté until soft.
2. Add chicken livers and cook until browned on the outside but still pink inside, about 5 minutes.
3. Transfer the liver mixture to a food processor, add cream, and blend until smooth.
4. Pass the mixture through a sieve for extra smoothness, then stir in the remaining butter.
5. Season with black pepper.
6. Refrigerate until firm, about 2 hours.
7. Serve chilled, garnished with fresh thyme.

Nutritional Info per Serving:

- Calories: 320
- Protein: 19g
- Carbohydrates: 5g
- Fat: 24g
- Fiber: 0g
- Sugar: 2g

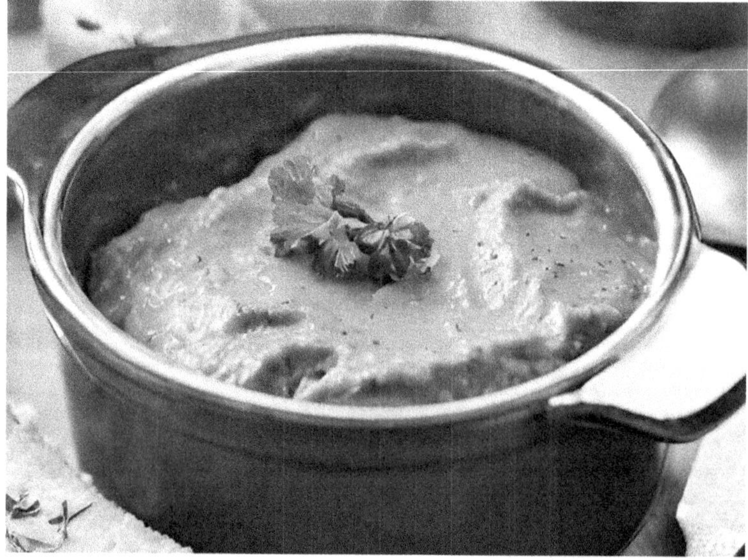

14. Buffalo Chicken Drumettes

Servings: 4
Cooking Time: 45 minutes
Ingredients:
- 2 pounds chicken drumettes
- 1/2 cup hot sauce
- 2 tablespoons butter, melted
- 1 teaspoon garlic powder
- Freshly ground black pepper

Instructions:
1. Preheat oven to 400°F (200°C).
2. In a bowl, combine hot sauce, melted butter, and garlic powder.
3. Toss the chicken drumettes in the sauce mixture until well coated.
4. Place on a baking sheet and sprinkle with black pepper.
5. Bake for 35 minutes, turning halfway through, until cooked through and crispy.
6. Serve hot.

Nutritional Info per Serving:
- Calories: 310
- Protein: 22g
- Carbohydrates: 0g
- Fat: 24g
- Fiber: 0g
- Sugar: 0g

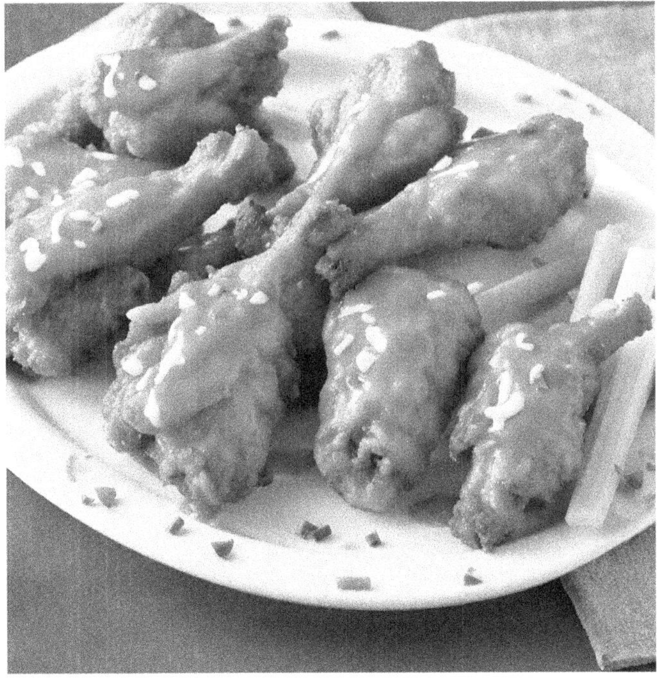

15. Roast Chicken with Herbs

Servings: 4

Cooking Time: 1 hour 30 minutes

Ingredients:

- 1 whole chicken (about 4 pounds)
- 2 tablespoons olive oil
- 1 tablespoon fresh rosemary, chopped
- 1 tablespoon fresh thyme, chopped
- 1 lemon, halved
- Freshly ground black pepper

Instructions:

1. Preheat oven to 375°F (190°C).
2. Rub the chicken with olive oil and sprinkle the chopped herbs all over.
3. Place lemon halves inside the chicken cavity.
4. Season the chicken with black pepper.
5. Roast in the oven for about 90 minutes, or until the juices run clear and a thermometer inserted into the thickest part of the thigh reads 165°F (75°C).
6. Let rest before carving. Serve hot.

Nutritional Info per Serving:

- Calories: 370
- Protein: 31g
- Carbohydrates: 1g
- Fat: 26g
- Fiber: 0g
- Sugar: 0g

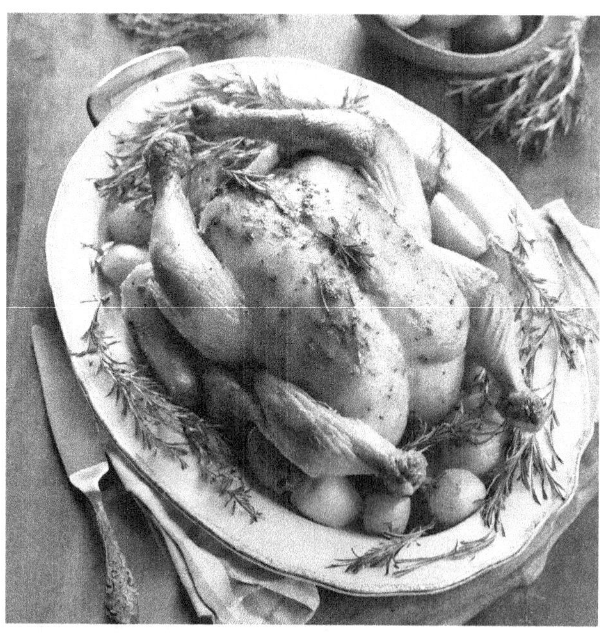

16. Chicken and Cabbage Soup

Servings: 6

Cooking Time: 1 hour

Ingredients:

- 1 pound chicken breasts, diced
- 1/2 head cabbage, chopped
- 1 onion, chopped
- 2 carrots, sliced
- 2 stalks celery, sliced
- 6 cups chicken broth
- 2 tablespoons olive oil
- 1 teaspoon thyme
- Freshly ground black pepper

Instructions:

1. In a large pot, heat olive oil over medium heat.
2. Add onion, carrots, and celery and sauté until softened.
3. Add diced chicken and cook until no longer pink.
4. Pour in chicken broth and bring to a boil.
5. Add cabbage and thyme, reduce heat, and simmer for 45 minutes.
6. Season with black pepper and serve hot.

Nutritional Info per Serving:

- Calories: 180
- Protein: 19g
- Carbohydrates: 7g
- Fat: 9g
- Fiber: 2g
- Sugar: 4g

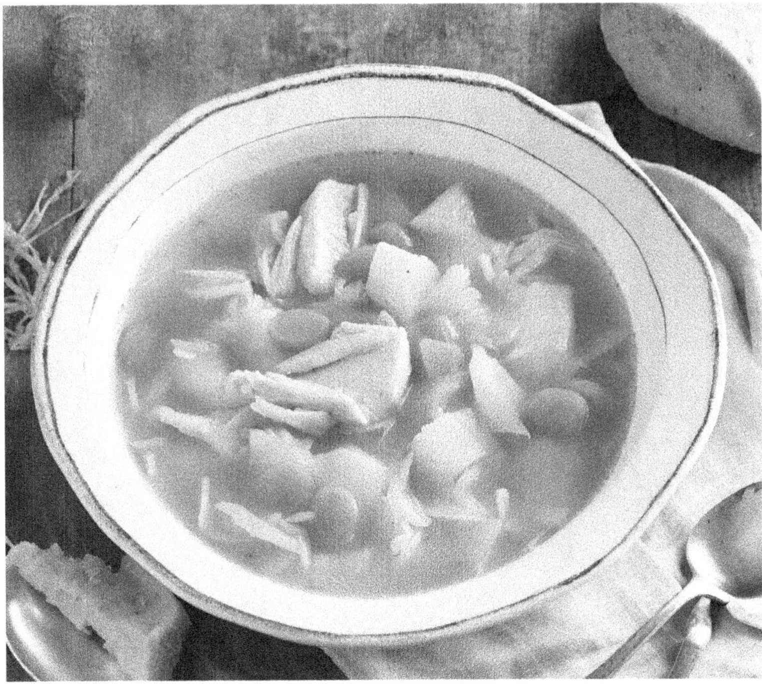

17. Chicken Bone Broth

Servings: 8
Cooking Time: 12 hours
Ingredients:

- 2 pounds chicken bones
- 1 onion, quartered
- 2 carrots, chopped
- 2 stalks celery, chopped
- 2 cloves garlic, smashed
- 1 tablespoon apple cider vinegar
- 12 cups water
- Fresh thyme
- Freshly ground black pepper

Instructions:

1. Place all ingredients in a large stockpot.
2. Bring to a boil, then reduce heat to a very low simmer.
3. Cover and simmer gently for 10-12 hours, skimming any foam that rises to the surface.
4. Strain the broth through a fine-mesh sieve, discarding solids.
5. Cool and store in the refrigerator or freezer. Season with black pepper when serving.

Nutritional Info per Serving:

- Calories: 40
- Protein: 6g
- Carbohydrates: 3g
- Fat: 1g
- Fiber: 1g
- Sugar: 1g

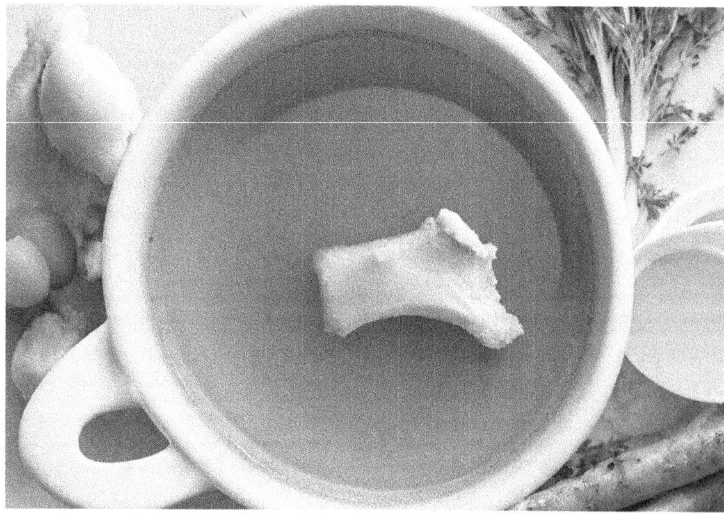

18. Balsamic Grilled Chicken Breast

Servings: 4

Cooking Time: 20 minutes

Ingredients:

- 4 chicken breasts
- 1/4 cup balsamic vinegar
- 2 tablespoons olive oil
- 1 teaspoon garlic powder
- Freshly ground black pepper

Instructions:

1. In a bowl, mix balsamic vinegar, olive oil, and garlic powder.
2. Marinate the chicken breasts in the mixture for at least 30 minutes.
3. Preheat grill to medium-high heat.
4. Grill chicken for 10 minutes per side, or until fully cooked.
5. Season with black pepper and serve hot.

Nutritional Info per Serving:

- Calories: 230
- Protein: 26g
- Carbohydrates: 3g
- Fat: 12g
- Fiber: 0g
- Sugar: 2g

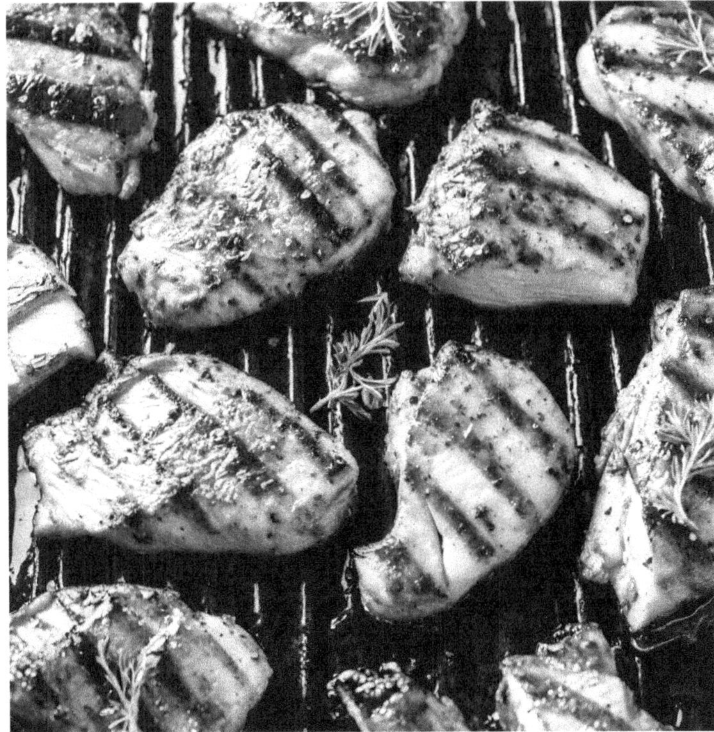

19. Smoked Turkey Drumsticks

Servings: 4
Cooking Time: 4 hours
Ingredients:

- 4 turkey drumsticks
- 1/4 cup apple cider vinegar
- 2 tablespoons smoked paprika
- 1 tablespoon garlic powder
- 1 tablespoon olive oil
- Freshly ground black pepper

Instructions:

1. Preheat your smoker to 225°F (107°C).
2. Mix the apple cider vinegar, smoked paprika, garlic powder, and olive oil in a bowl. Rub this mixture all over the turkey drumsticks.
3. Place the drumsticks in the smoker and cook for about 4 hours, or until the meat is tender and reaches an internal temperature of 165°F (74°C).
4. Season with black pepper and serve hot.

Nutritional Info per Serving:

- Calories: 310
- Protein: 44g
- Carbohydrates: 2g
- Fat: 14g
- Fiber: 0g
- Sugar: 1g

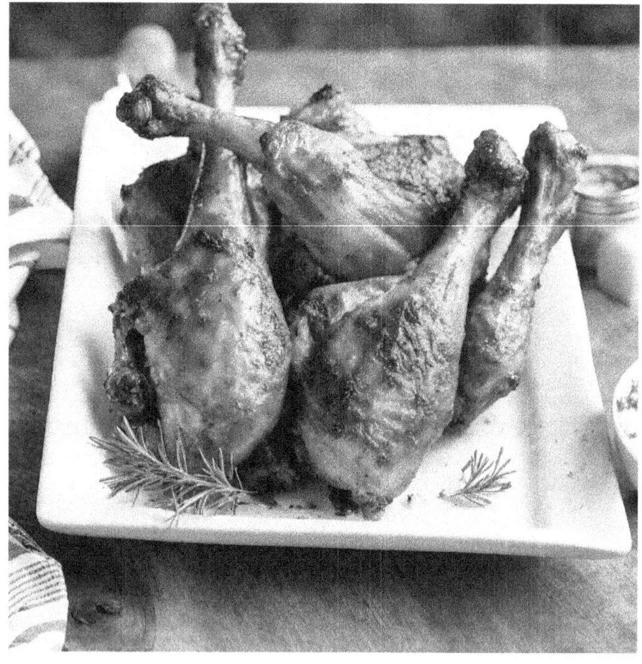

20. Turkey and Egg Breakfast Casserole

Servings: 6
Cooking Time: 1 hour
Ingredients:

- 6 eggs
- 1 pound ground turkey
- 1 cup diced bell peppers
- 1 cup chopped spinach
- 1 onion, diced
- 1/2 cup milk
- 1 tablespoon olive oil
- Freshly ground black pepper
- Fresh herbs (such as parsley or thyme), for garnish

Instructions:

1. Preheat oven to 350°F (175°C).
2. Heat olive oil in a skillet over medium heat. Add ground turkey and onion, cooking until turkey is browned and onions are soft.
3. In a large bowl, whisk together eggs and milk. Stir in cooked turkey, bell peppers, and spinach.
4. Pour the mixture into a greased baking dish.
5. Bake for 45 minutes, or until the eggs are set and the top is lightly golden.
6. Season with black pepper and garnish with fresh herbs before serving.

Nutritional Info per Serving:

- Calories: 240
- Protein: 27g
- Carbohydrates: 6g
- Fat: 12g
- Fiber: 1g
- Sugar: 3g

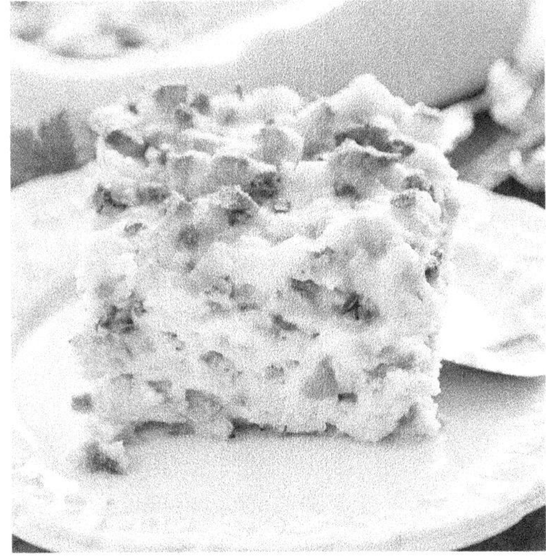

21. Spicy Turkey Chili
Servings: 6
Cooking Time: 1 hour
Ingredients:
- 1 pound ground turkey
- 1 can (15 oz) diced tomatoes
- 1 can (15 oz) kidney beans, drained and rinsed
- 1 onion, chopped
- 1 bell pepper, chopped
- 2 cloves garlic, minced
- 2 tablespoons chili powder
- 1 teaspoon cumin
- 1 tablespoon olive oil
- Freshly ground black pepper
- Fresh cilantro, for garnish

Instructions:
1. Heat olive oil in a large pot over medium heat. Add onion, bell pepper, and garlic and sauté until soft.
2. Add ground turkey and cook until browned.
3. Stir in chili powder and cumin, cooking for another minute.
4. Add diced tomatoes and kidney beans. Bring to a boil, then reduce heat and simmer for 45 minutes.
5. Season with black pepper and garnish with fresh cilantro before serving.

Nutritional Info per Serving:
- Calories: 270
- Protein: 22g
- Carbohydrates: 19g
- Fat: 12g
- Fiber: 5g
- Sugar: 4g

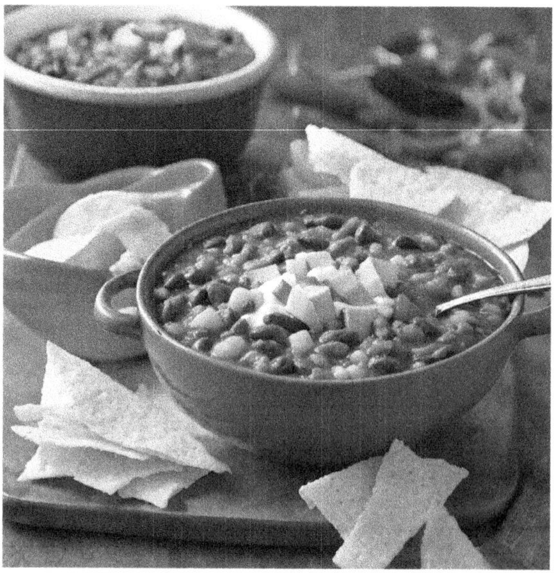

22. Turkey Bacon Wrapped Asparagus

Servings: 4
Cooking Time: 20 minutes
Ingredients:

- 16 asparagus spears, trimmed
- 8 slices turkey bacon
- 1 tablespoon olive oil
- Freshly ground black pepper

Instructions:

1. Preheat oven to 400°F (200°C).
2. Wrap each asparagus spear with half a slice of turkey bacon, securing with a toothpick if necessary.
3. Arrange on a baking sheet and drizzle with olive oil.
4. Roast in the oven for 15-20 minutes, or until the bacon is crispy and asparagus is tender.
5. Season with black pepper and serve hot.

Nutritional Info per Serving:

- Calories: 150
- Protein: 10g
- Carbohydrates: 2g
- Fat: 11g
- Fiber: 1g
- Sugar: 1g

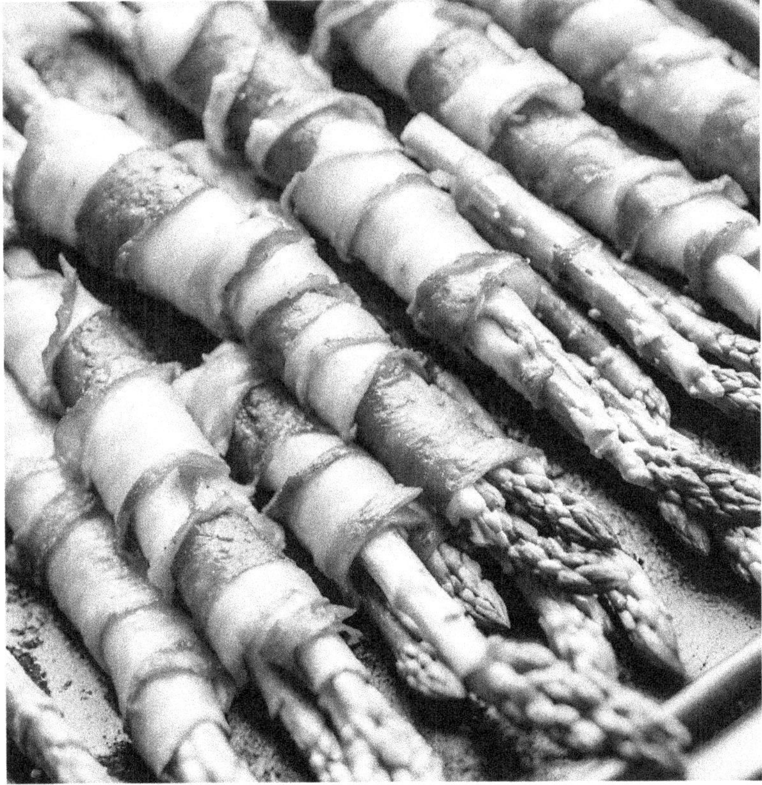

23. Baked Turkey Wings

Servings: 4
Cooking Time: 1 hour 20 minutes
Ingredients:

- 4 turkey wings, split at the joints
- 2 tablespoons olive oil
- 1 teaspoon smoked paprika
- 1 teaspoon garlic powder
- Freshly ground black pepper

Instructions:

1. Preheat oven to 375°F (190°C).
2. Rub the turkey wings with olive oil, smoked paprika, and garlic powder.
3. Place on a baking sheet and season with black pepper.
4. Bake for 1 hour and 20 minutes, or until the skin is crispy and the meat is tender and fully cooked.

Nutritional Info per Serving:

- Calories: 420
- Protein: 35g
- Carbohydrates: 0g
- Fat: 30g
- Fiber: 0g
- Sugar: 0g

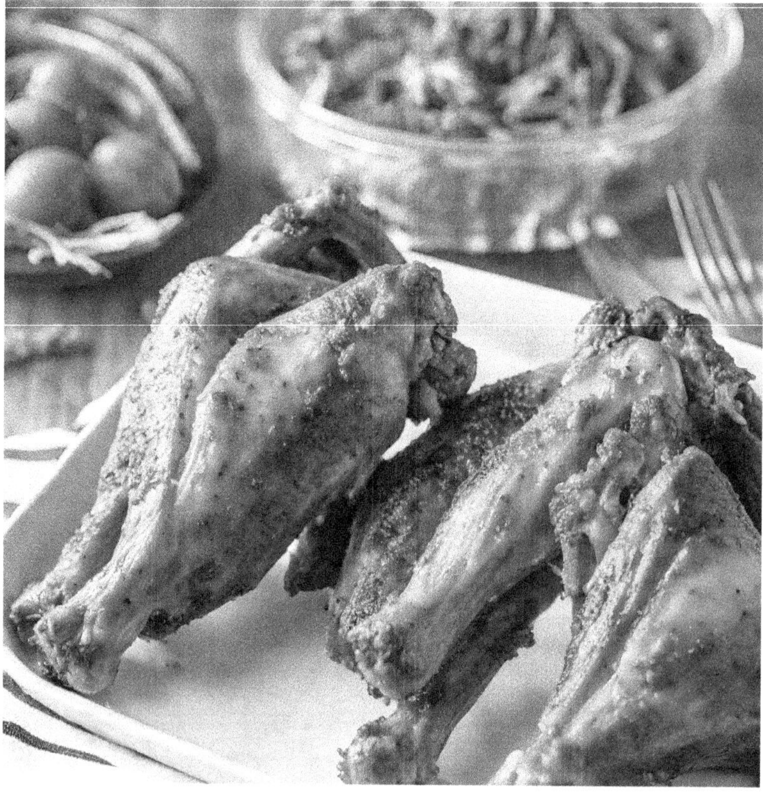

24. Turkey and Kale Stir-Fry

Servings: 4

Cooking Time: 30 minutes

Ingredients:

- 1 pound turkey breast, sliced thinly
- 2 cups kale, chopped
- 1 red bell pepper, sliced
- 1 onion, sliced
- 2 cloves garlic, minced
- 2 tablespoons soy sauce (or tamari for gluten-free option)
- 1 tablespoon sesame oil
- Freshly ground black pepper
- 1 tablespoon olive oil

Instructions:

1. Heat olive oil in a large skillet over medium-high heat.
2. Add turkey slices and cook until browned, about 5-6 minutes.
3. Add garlic, onion, and bell pepper and sauté for another 5 minutes.
4. Add kale and cook until it starts to wilt, about 3-4 minutes.
5. Stir in soy sauce and sesame oil, mixing well.
6. Season with black pepper and cook for another 2 minutes.
7. Serve hot.

Nutritional Info per Serving:

- Calories: 220
- Protein: 27g
- Carbohydrates: 8g
- Fat: 9g
- Fiber: 2g
- Sugar: 3g

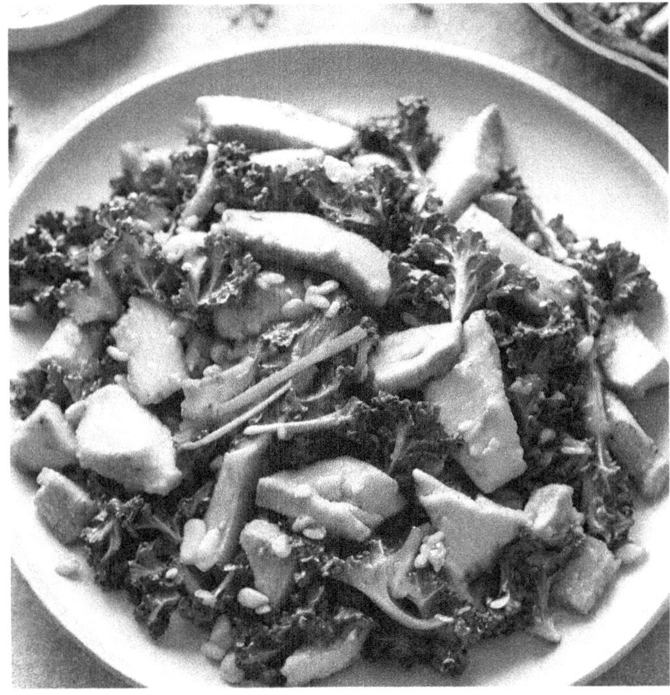

25. Herb-Roasted Turkey Breast

Servings: 6

Cooking Time: 1 hour 30 minutes

Ingredients:

- 3 pounds turkey breast
- 2 tablespoons olive oil
- 1 tablespoon chopped fresh rosemary
- 1 tablespoon chopped fresh thyme
- 1 tablespoon chopped fresh sage
- Freshly ground black pepper

Instructions:

1. Preheat oven to 325°F (165°C).
2. Rub the turkey breast with olive oil and then coat with the chopped herbs.
3. Place in a roasting pan and season generously with black pepper.
4. Roast in the preheated oven for about 1 hour and 30 minutes, or until a thermometer inserted into the thickest part of the breast reads 165°F (74°C).
5. Let the turkey rest for 10 minutes before slicing. Serve hot.

Nutritional Info per Serving:

- Calories: 250
- Protein: 51g
- Carbohydrates: 0g
- Fat: 5g
- Fiber: 0g
- Sugar: 0g

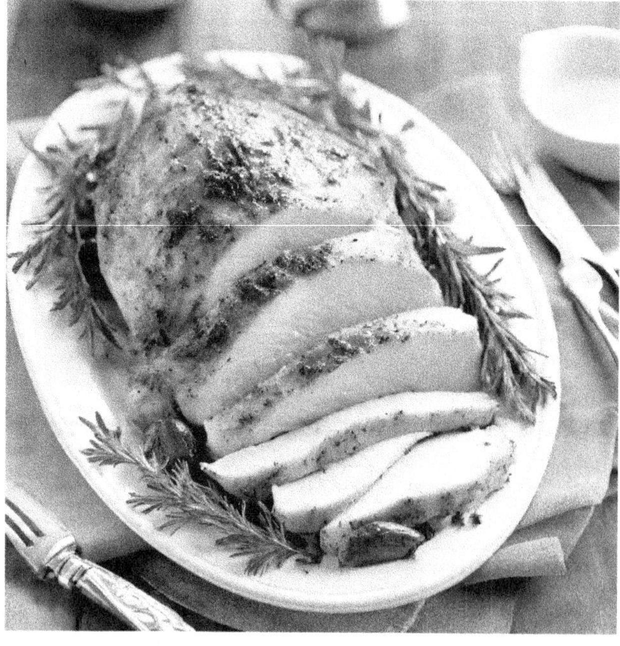

Beef & Pork

1. Argentinean Beef Skewers with Chimichurri Sauce
Servings: 4
Cooking Time: 20 minutes (plus marinating time)
Ingredients:
- 1.5 pounds beef sirloin, cut into cubes
- 2 tablespoons olive oil
- **For the Chimichurri Sauce:**
    - 1 cup fresh parsley, chopped
    - 1/4 cup olive oil
    - 2 tablespoons red wine vinegar
    - 3 garlic cloves, minced
    - 1 teaspoon chili flakes
    - 1 teaspoon dried oregano

Instructions:
1. Marinate the beef cubes in olive oil and set aside for at least 30 minutes.
2. Preheat grill to medium-high heat.
3. Thread the beef cubes onto skewers.
4. Grill for 10-12 minutes, turning occasionally, until cooked to your liking.
5. For the chimichurri sauce, combine parsley, olive oil, vinegar, garlic, chili flakes, and oregano in a bowl. Mix well.
6. Serve the skewers drizzled with chimichurri sauce.

Nutritional Info per Serving:
- Calories: 480
- Protein: 40g
- Carbohydrates: 2g
- Fat: 34g
- Fiber: 1g
- Sugar: 0g

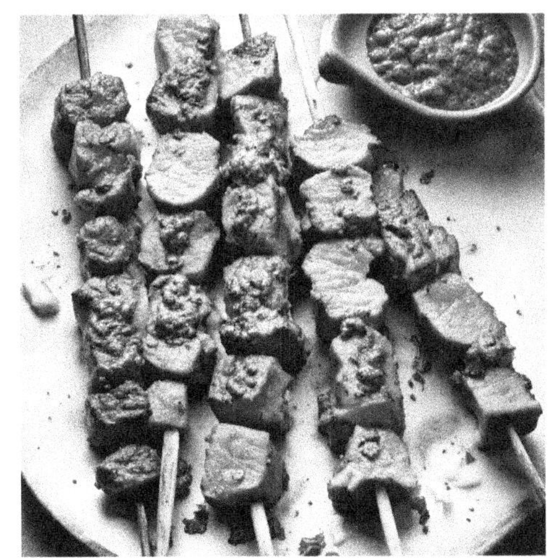

2. Pork Back Ribs with Smoky Rub

Servings: 4
Cooking Time: 3 hours
Ingredients:

- 2 pounds pork back ribs
- 2 tablespoons smoked paprika
- 1 tablespoon garlic powder
- 1 tablespoon onion powder
- 2 teaspoons cumin
- 1 tablespoon olive oil

Instructions:

1. Preheat your oven to 275°F (135°C).
2. Combine smoked paprika, garlic powder, onion powder, and cumin in a bowl.
3. Rub the ribs with olive oil and then coat with the spice mixture.
4. Place ribs on a baking sheet, cover with foil, and bake for about 3 hours or until tender.
5. Optional: Finish on a grill for 5 minutes per side to char slightly.
6. Serve hot.

Nutritional Info per Serving:

- Calories: 560
- Protein: 35g
- Carbohydrates: 3g
- Fat: 44g
- Fiber: 1g
- Sugar: 0g

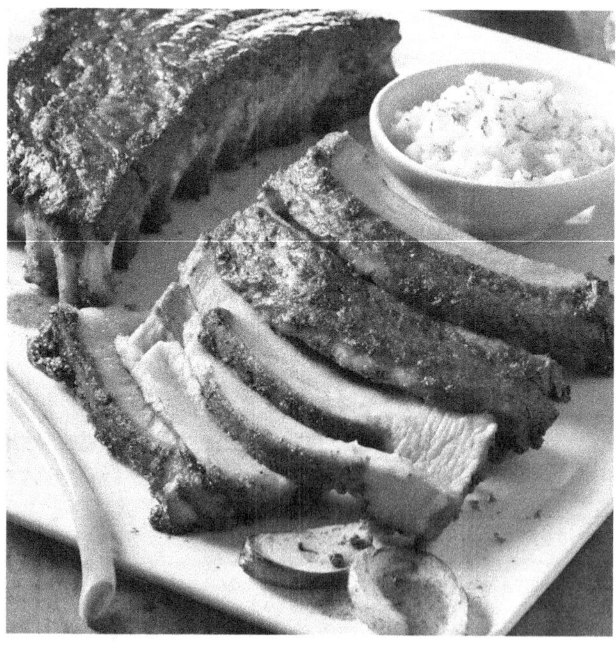

3. Cured Pork Loin Carpaccio

Servings: 4

Cooking Time: 10 minutes (plus curing time)

Ingredients:

- 1 pound pork loin, thinly sliced
- 1/4 cup coarse sea salt
- 1/4 cup sugar
- 1 tablespoon crushed juniper berries
- 1 tablespoon olive oil
- Fresh herbs for garnish

Instructions:

1. Combine sea salt, sugar, and crushed juniper berries in a bowl.
2. Coat the pork loin slices with the curing mixture and refrigerate for at least 12 hours.
3. Rinse off the cure under cold water and pat dry.
4. Arrange the slices on a plate, drizzle with olive oil, and garnish with fresh herbs.
5. Serve immediately.

Nutritional Info per Serving:

- Calories: 230
- Protein: 25g
- Carbohydrates: 12g
- Fat: 9g
- Fiber: 0g
- Sugar: 12g

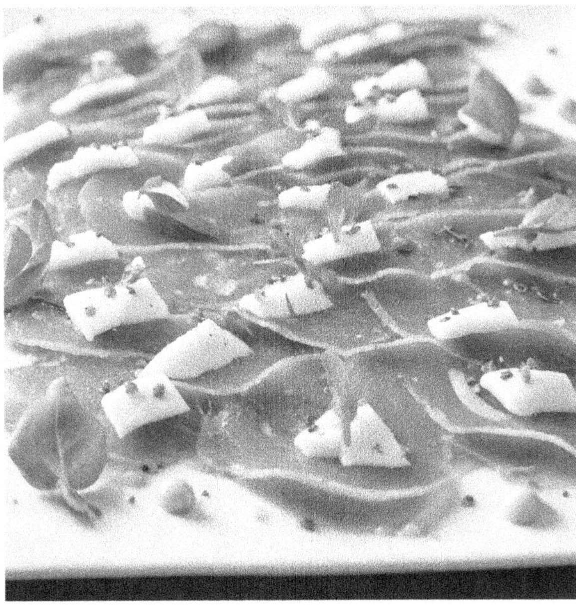

4. Beef and Pork Goulash

Servings: 6

Cooking Time: 2 hours

Ingredients:

- 1 pound beef chuck, cubed
- 1 pound pork shoulder, cubed
- 1 onion, chopped
- 2 cloves garlic, minced
- 1 tablespoon smoked paprika
- 1 can (14 oz) diced tomatoes
- 4 cups beef broth
- 1 tablespoon olive oil
- Fresh herbs (such as parsley), for garnish

Instructions:

1. Heat olive oil in a large pot over medium heat.
2. Add onion and garlic, sautéing until translucent.
3. Add beef and pork cubes, browning on all sides.
4. Stir in smoked paprika, then add tomatoes and beef broth.
5. Bring to a boil, reduce heat to low, and simmer covered for 1.5 hours, until meat is tender.
6. Garnish with fresh herbs and serve hot.

Nutritional Info per Serving:

- Calories: 400
- Protein: 38g
- Carbohydrates: 6g
- Fat: 24g
- Fiber: 1g
- Sugar: 3g

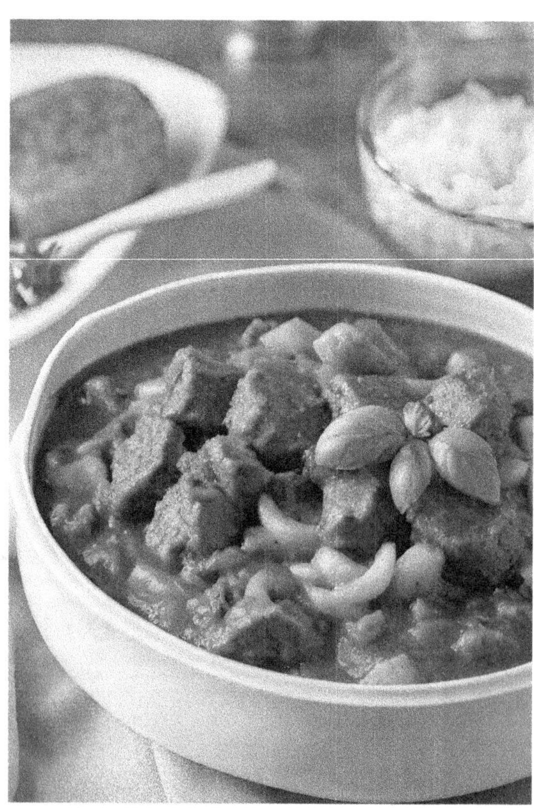

5. Grilled Beef and Pork Burgers

Servings: 4
Cooking Time: 20 minutes
Ingredients:

- 1/2 pound ground beef
- 1/2 pound ground pork
- 1/4 cup minced onion
- 1 egg, beaten
- 1 tablespoon olive oil
- Freshly ground black pepper

Instructions:

1. In a bowl, mix ground beef, ground pork, onion, and egg.
2. Form the mixture into 4 patties.
3. Preheat grill to medium-high.
4. Brush the grill grate with olive oil and grill patties for about 10 minutes per side, or until fully cooked.
5. Season with black pepper and serve on buns or lettuce wraps.

Nutritional Info per Serving:

- Calories: 350
- Protein: 28g
- Carbohydrates: 2g
- Fat: 25g
- Fiber: 0g
- Sugar: 1g

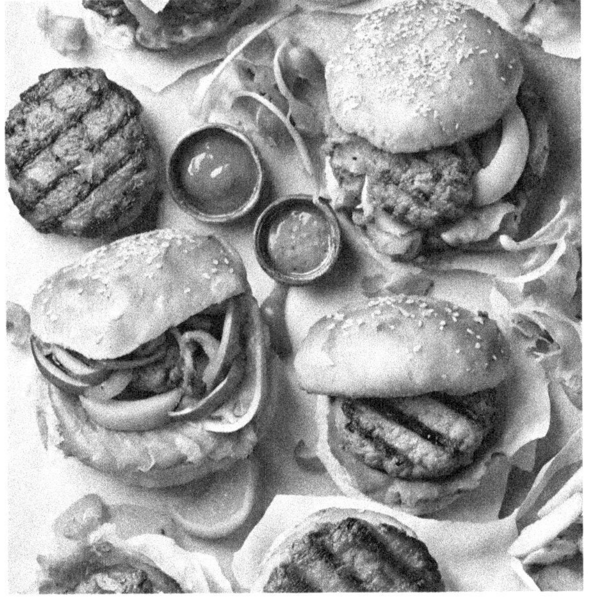

6. Mini Meatballs (Beef and Pork)

Servings: 4
Cooking Time: 30 minutes
Ingredients:

- 1/2 pound ground beef
- 1/2 pound ground pork
- 1/4 cup minced onion
- 1 egg, beaten
- 1/4 cup almond flour
- 1 tablespoon garlic powder
- 1 tablespoon dried oregano
- 1 tablespoon olive oil

Instructions:

1. Preheat oven to 375°F (190°C).
2. In a bowl, combine ground beef, ground pork, onion, egg, almond flour, garlic powder, and oregano.
3. Form into small meatballs, approximately 1 inch in diameter.
4. Place meatballs on a baking sheet lined with parchment paper.
5. Bake for 20-25 minutes, or until browned and cooked through.
6. Drizzle with olive oil before serving.

Nutritional Info per Serving:

- Calories: 320
- Protein: 22g
- Carbohydrates: 4g
- Fat: 24g
- Fiber: 1g
- Sugar: 1g

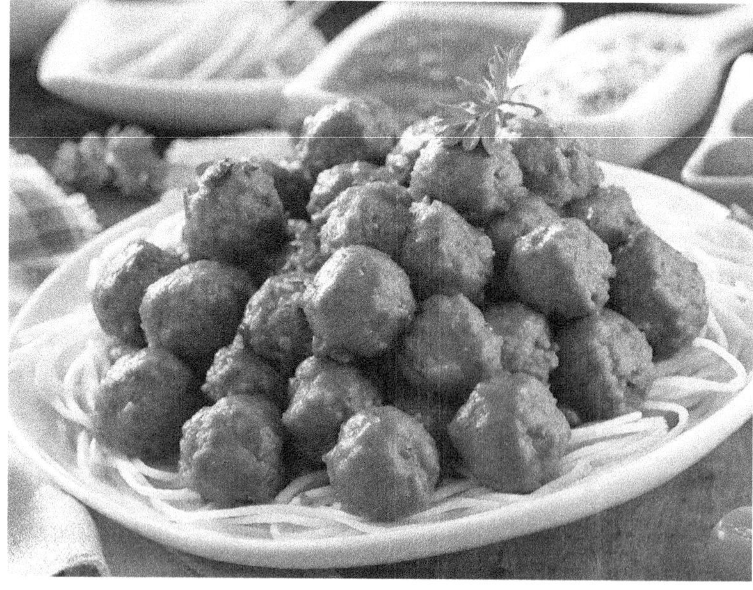

7. Beef and Pork Ragout

Servings: 6

Cooking Time: 2 hours 30 minutes

Ingredients:

- 1/2 pound ground beef
- 1/2 pound ground pork
- 1 onion, chopped
- 2 cloves garlic, minced
- 1 can (14 oz) crushed tomatoes
- 2 cups beef broth
- 1 tablespoon dried basil
- 1 tablespoon dried thyme
- 1 tablespoon olive oil

Instructions:

1. Heat olive oil in a large pot over medium heat.
2. Add onion and garlic and sauté until soft.
3. Add ground beef and pork, and cook until browned.
4. Stir in crushed tomatoes, beef broth, basil, and thyme.
5. Bring to a boil, then reduce heat and simmer for 2 hours.
6. Serve hot, garnished with fresh herbs if desired.

Nutritional Info per Serving:

- Calories: 350
- Protein: 25g
- Carbohydrates: 8g
- Fat: 24g
- Fiber: 2g
- Sugar: 4g

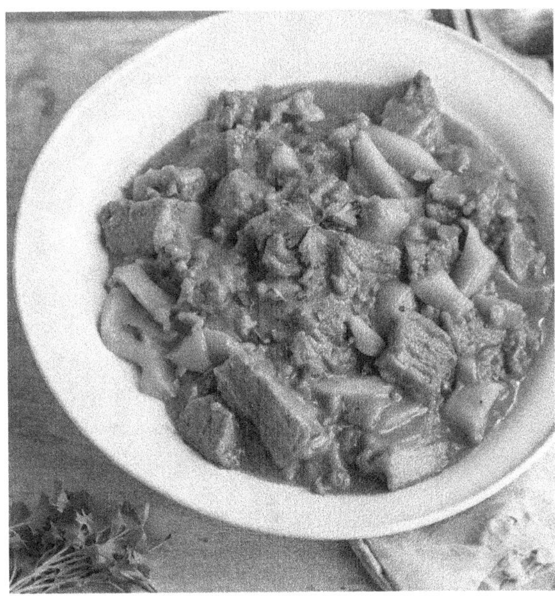

8. Stuffed Peppers with Beef and Pork

Servings: 4
Cooking Time: 1 hour
Ingredients:

- 4 bell peppers, tops cut off and seeds removed
- 1/2 pound ground beef
- 1/2 pound ground pork
- 1 cup cooked rice
- 1 onion, finely chopped
- 1 egg, beaten
- 1 can (14 oz) crushed tomatoes
- 1 tablespoon dried marjoram
- 1 tablespoon olive oil

Instructions:

1. Preheat oven to 350°F (175°C).
2. In a skillet, heat olive oil over medium heat. Add onion and cook until translucent.
3. Add ground beef and pork, cooking until browned.
4. Remove from heat and mix in cooked rice, egg, and marjoram.
5. Stuff the mixture into the bell peppers and place them in a baking dish.
6. Pour crushed tomatoes over the peppers.
7. Bake for 45 minutes, or until the peppers are tender.

Nutritional Info per Serving:

- Calories: 400
- Protein: 26g
- Carbohydrates: 22g
- Fat: 22g
- Fiber: 4g
- Sugar: 8g

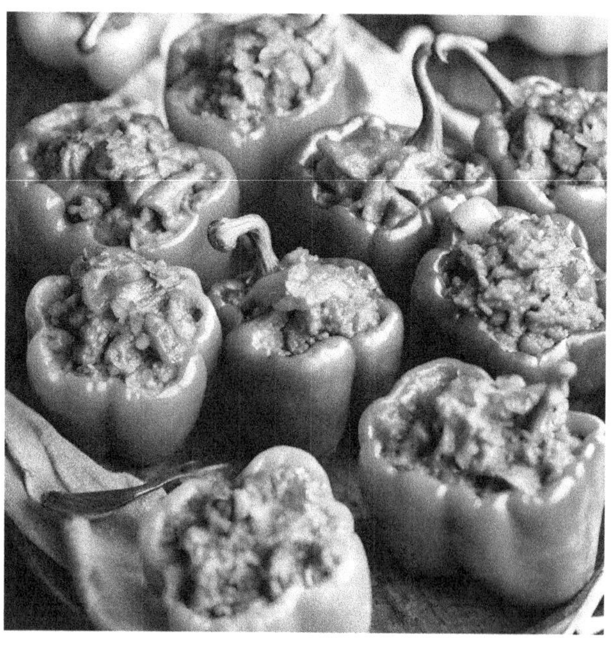

9. Beef and Pork Chili

Servings: 6

Cooking Time: 1 hour 20 minutes

Ingredients:

- 1/2 pound ground beef
- 1/2 pound ground pork
- 1 onion, chopped
- 2 cloves garlic, minced
- 1 can (15 oz) kidney beans, drained and rinsed
- 1 can (28 oz) diced tomatoes
- 2 tablespoons chili powder
- 1 teaspoon cumin
- 1 tablespoon olive oil

Instructions:

1. Heat olive oil in a large pot over medium heat.
2. Add onion and garlic, sautéing until soft.
3. Add ground beef and pork, cooking until browned.
4. Stir in diced tomatoes, kidney beans, chili powder, and cumin.
5. Bring to a boil, then reduce heat and simmer for 1 hour.
6. Serve hot, garnished with fresh cilantro if desired.

Nutritional Info per Serving:

- Calories: 340
- Protein: 24g
- Carbohydrates: 18g
- Fat: 19g
- Fiber: 6g
- Sugar: 5g

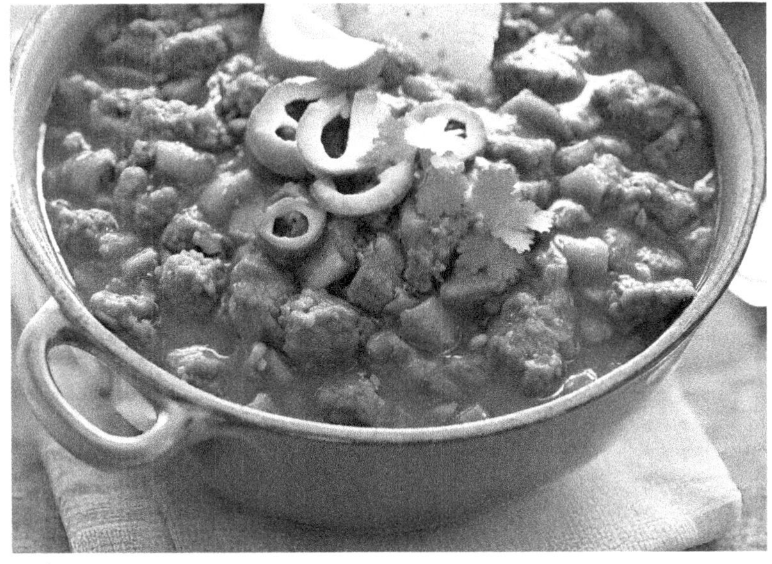

10. Meatloaf with Ground Beef and Pork

Servings: 6

Cooking Time: 1 hour 15 minutes

Ingredients:

- 1/2 pound ground beef
- 1/2 pound ground pork
- 1 cup almond flour
- 1 onion, finely chopped
- 2 cloves garlic, minced
- 1 egg, beaten
- 1/2 cup crushed tomatoes
- 1 tablespoon dried parsley
- 1 tablespoon olive oil

Instructions:

1. Preheat oven to 375°F (190°C).
2. In a large bowl, mix together ground beef, ground pork, almond flour, onion, garlic, egg, and parsley.
3. Shape the mixture into a loaf and place it in a greased baking pan.
4. Brush the top of the loaf with crushed tomatoes.
5. Bake in the preheated oven for 1 hour or until the meatloaf is cooked through.
6. Let it rest for 10 minutes before slicing. Drizzle with olive oil before serving.

Nutritional Info per Serving:

- Calories: 330
- Protein: 22g
- Carbohydrates: 9g
- Fat: 23g
- Fiber: 3g
- Sugar: 3g

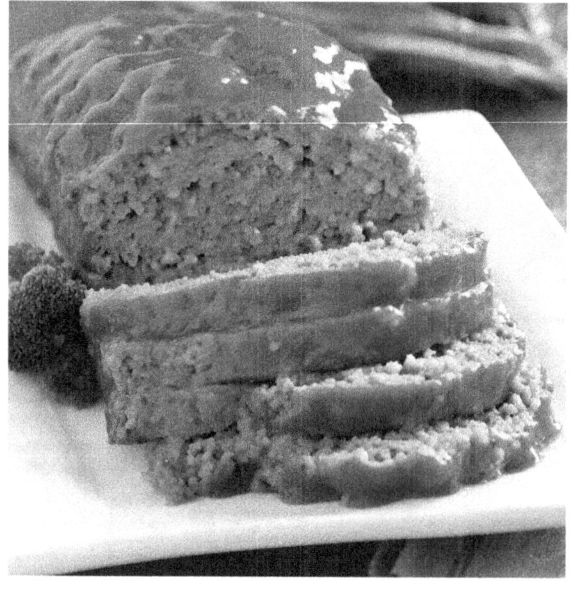

11. Pork and Fennel Sausage Patties

Servings: 4

Cooking Time: 20 minutes

Ingredients:

- 1 pound ground pork
- 1 fennel bulb, finely chopped
- 1 teaspoon fennel seeds
- 1 egg
- 1 tablespoon olive oil

Instructions:

1. In a bowl, combine ground pork, chopped fennel bulb, fennel seeds, and egg. Mix well.
2. Form the mixture into small patties.
3. Heat olive oil in a skillet over medium heat.
4. Cook the patties for about 4-5 minutes on each side or until fully cooked.
5. Serve hot.

Nutritional Info per Serving:

- Calories: 300
- Protein: 20g
- Carbohydrates: 5g
- Fat: 22g
- Fiber: 2g
- Sugar: 2g

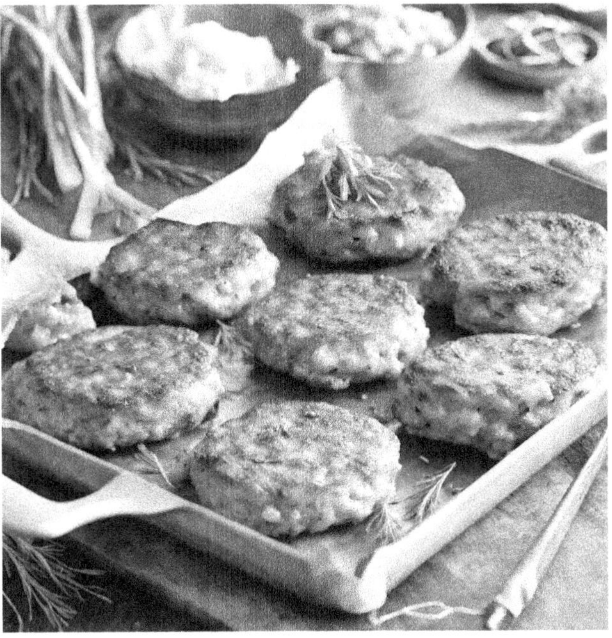

12. Pork and Parsnip Soup

Servings: 6
Cooking Time: 1 hour
Ingredients:

- 1 pound pork shoulder, cut into cubes
- 3 parsnips, peeled and chopped
- 1 onion, chopped
- 6 cups chicken broth
- 1 tablespoon olive oil
- 1 teaspoon thyme

Instructions:

1. Heat olive oil in a large pot over medium heat.
2. Add onion and sauté until translucent.
3. Add pork cubes and brown all sides.
4. Pour in chicken broth and bring to a boil.
5. Add parsnips and thyme. Reduce heat and simmer for about 45 minutes or until pork is tender.
6. Serve hot.

Nutritional Info per Serving:

- Calories: 220
- Protein: 18g
- Carbohydrates: 10g
- Fat: 11g
- Fiber: 3g
- Sugar: 4g

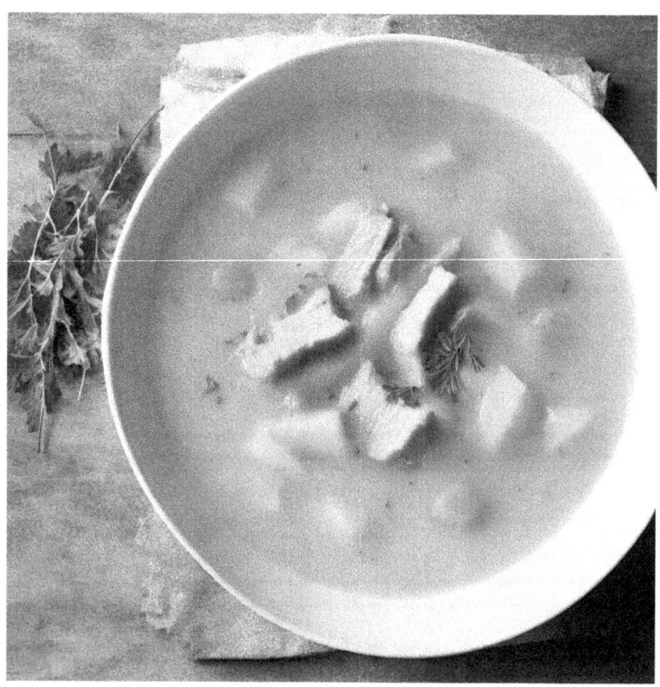

13. Grilled Pork Loin with Garlic and Herbs

Servings: 4
Cooking Time: 1 hour
Ingredients:

- 2 pounds pork loin
- 4 cloves garlic, minced
- 1 tablespoon rosemary, minced
- 1 tablespoon thyme, minced
- 1 tablespoon olive oil

Instructions:

1. Preheat your grill to medium-high heat.
2. Mix garlic, rosemary, thyme, and olive oil in a bowl. Rub this mixture all over the pork loin.
3. Grill the pork loin for about 50-60 minutes, turning occasionally, until the internal temperature reaches 145°F (63°C).
4. Let rest for 10 minutes before slicing. Serve hot.

Nutritional Info per Serving:

- Calories: 340
- Protein: 50g
- Carbohydrates: 1g
- Fat: 15g
- Fiber: 0g
- Sugar: 0g

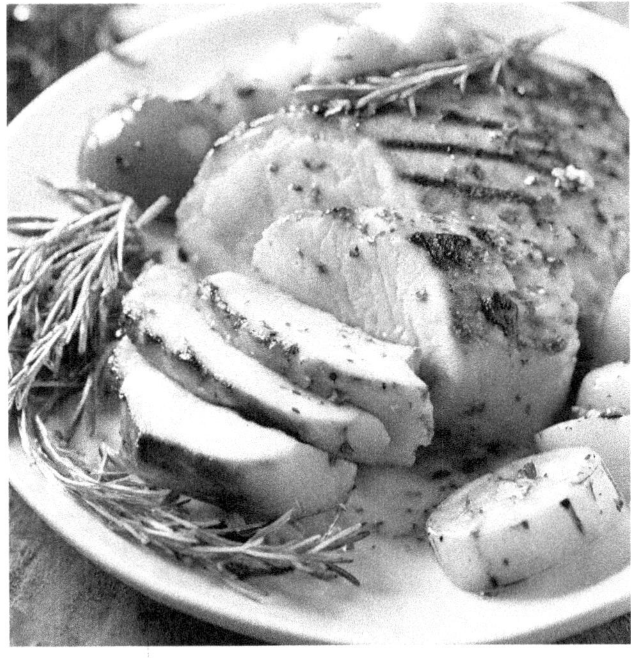

14. Pork Belly with Sea Salt and Rosemary
Servings: 4
Cooking Time: 3 hours
Ingredients:
- 2 pounds pork belly
- 1 tablespoon sea salt
- 1 tablespoon rosemary, minced
- 1 tablespoon olive oil

Instructions:
1. Preheat oven to 275°F (135°C).
2. Score the skin of the pork belly with a sharp knife. Rub with olive oil, then season with sea salt and Rosemary
3. Place pork belly skin-side up in a roasting pan.
4. Roast in the preheated oven for about 3 hours or until the meat is very tender and the skin is crisp.
5. Let rest for 10 minutes before slicing. Serve hot.

Nutritional Info per Serving:
- Calories: 580
- Protein: 14g
- Carbohydrates:0g
- Fat: 58g
- Fiber: 0g
- Sugar: 0g

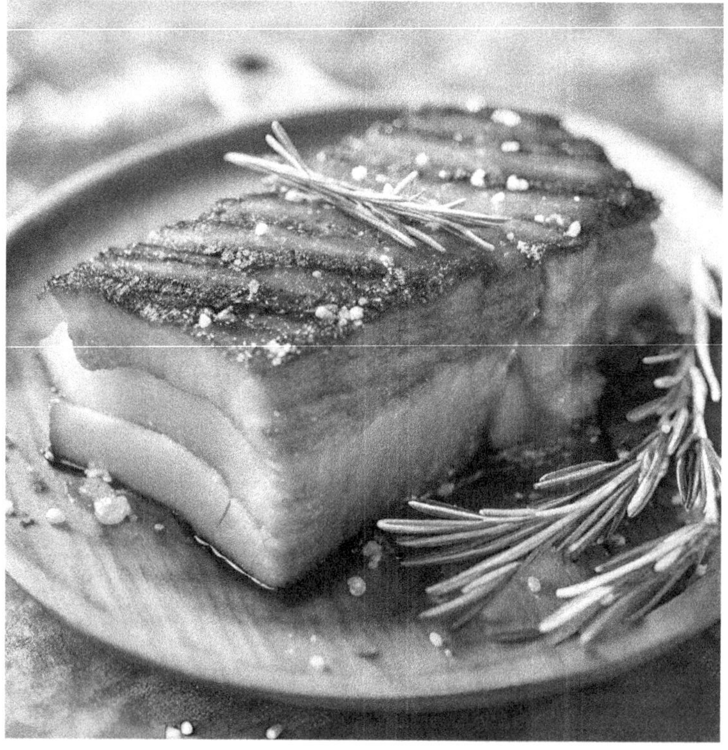

15. Spicy Pork Rinds

Servings: 4
Cooking Time: 1 hour (plus drying time)
Ingredients:

- 1 pound pork skin, cut into 2-inch pieces
- 2 tablespoons cayenne pepper
- 1 tablespoon smoked paprika
- 1 tablespoon olive oil

Instructions:

1. Preheat oven to 200°F (93°C).
2. Boil pork skin in water for 1 hour until tender. Drain and pat dry.
3. Place pork skin pieces on a baking sheet and bake for 4-6 hours or until completely dried out.
4. Increase oven temperature to 400°F (200°C).
5. Toss dried pork skins with olive oil, cayenne pepper, and smoked paprika.
6. Bake for another 10-15 minutes or until puffed and crispy.
7. Serve hot.

Nutritional Info per Serving:

- Calories: 500
- Protein: 28g
- Carbohydrates: 0g
- Fat: 44g
- Fiber: 0g
- Sugar: 0g

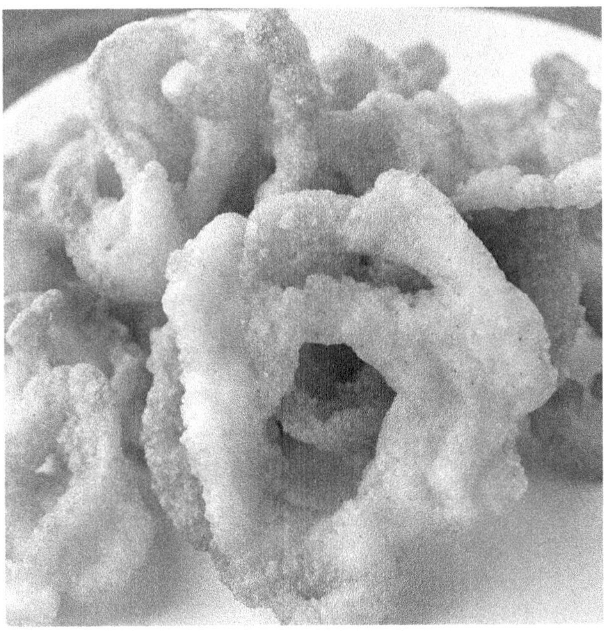

16. Herb-Stuffed Pork Tenderloin

Servings: 4
Cooking Time: 45 minutes
Ingredients:

- 2 pounds pork tenderloin
- 1/4 cup fresh parsley, chopped
- 1/4 cup fresh sage, chopped
- 2 cloves garlic, minced
- 1 tablespoon olive oil

Instructions:

1. Preheat oven to 375°F (190°C).
2. Make a lengthwise cut along the center of the pork tenderloin to create a pocket.
3. Mix parsley, sage, and garlic. Stuff this mixture into the pork pocket.
4. Tie the tenderloin with kitchen string to secure the stuffing.
5. Rub the outside with olive oil.
6. Roast in the preheated oven for about 35-40 minutes, or until the internal temperature reaches 145°F (63°C).
7. Let rest for 10 minutes before slicing. Serve hot.

Nutritional Info per Serving:

- Calories: 310
- Protein: 48g
- Carbohydrates: 1g
- Fat: 12g
- Fiber: 0g
- Sugar: 0g

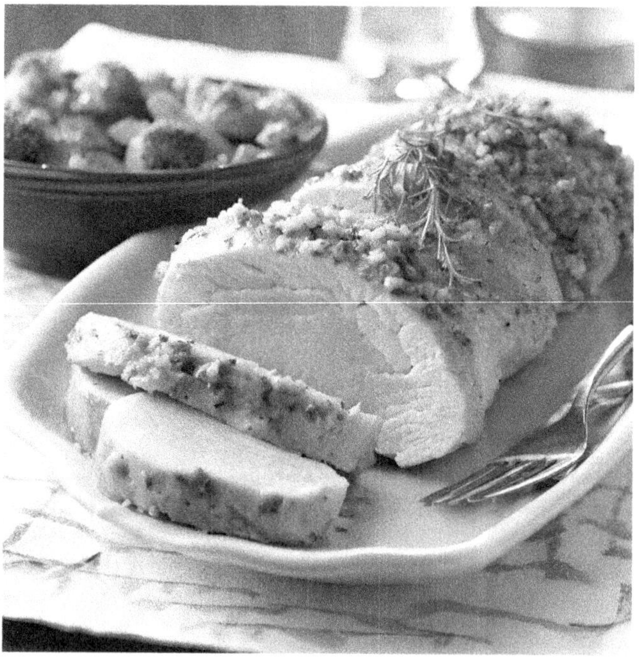

17. Pulled Pork with Cabbage Slaw

Servings: 6

Cooking Time: 8 hours

Ingredients:

- 3 pounds pork shoulder
- 1 cup barbecue sauce
- 1/2 head cabbage, shredded
- 1/4 cup apple cider vinegar
- 1 tablespoon olive oil
- 1 teaspoon mustard seeds

Instructions:

1. Place pork shoulder in a slow cooker and cover with barbecue sauce.
2. Cook on low for 8 hours or until the pork is very tender.
3. Remove pork, shred with forks, and mix back with the sauce in the cooker.
4. For the slaw, mix cabbage with apple cider vinegar, olive oil, and mustard seeds.
5. Serve the pulled pork topped with cabbage slaw.

Nutritional Info per Serving:

- Calories: 580
- Protein: 48g
- Carbohydrates: 15g
- Fat: 36g
- Fiber: 3g
- Sugar: 12g

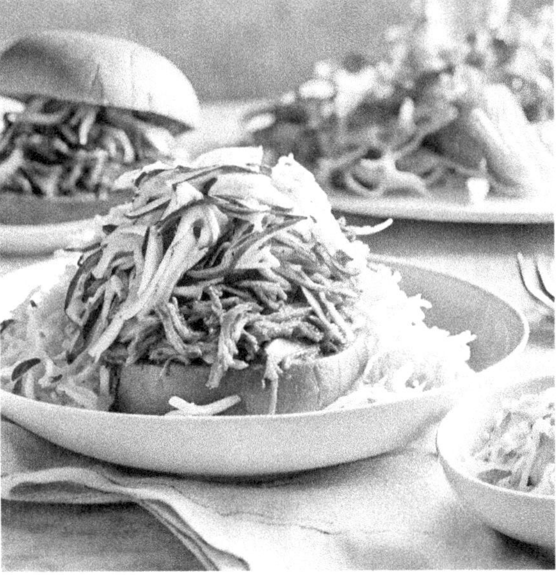

18. Italian Beef Stew

Servings: 6

Cooking Time: 2 hours 30 minutes

Ingredients:

- 2 pounds beef chuck, cut into cubes
- 1 onion, chopped
- 2 carrots, chopped
- 2 celery stalks, chopped
- 4 garlic cloves, minced
- 1 can (28 oz) crushed tomatoes
- 2 cups beef broth
- 1 cup red wine
- 1 tablespoon dried basil
- 1 tablespoon dried oregano
- 1 tablespoon olive oil

Instructions:

1. Heat olive oil in a large pot over medium-high heat.
2. Brown the beef cubes on all sides and set aside.
3. In the same pot, sauté onion, carrots, celery, and garlic until onion is translucent.
4. Add the browned beef back into the pot along with crushed tomatoes, beef broth, red wine, basil, and oregano.
5. Bring to a boil, then reduce heat and simmer, covered, for about 2 hours, until the beef is tender.
6. Serve hot, garnished with fresh herbs if desired.

Nutritional Info per Serving:

- Calories: 420
- Protein: 35g
- Carbohydrates: 15g
- Fat: 20g
- Fiber: 3g
- Sugar: 8g

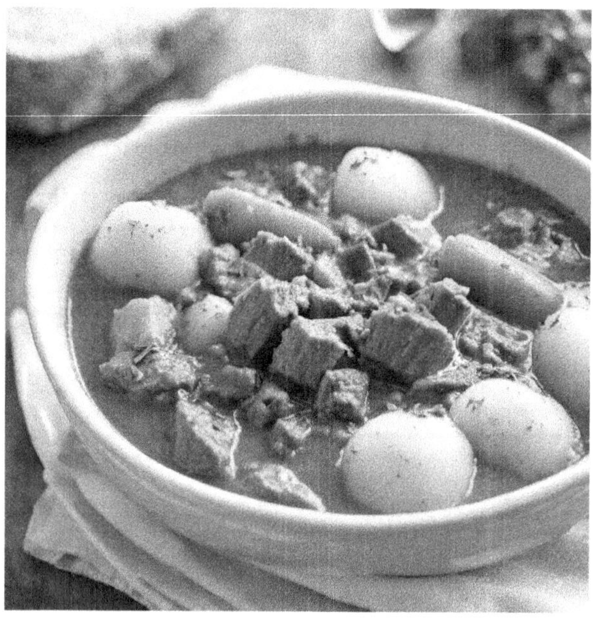

19. Balsamic Glazed Beef Ribs

Servings: 4

Cooking Time: 3 hours

Ingredients:

- 4 pounds beef ribs
- 1 cup balsamic vinegar
- 2 tablespoons honey
- 1 tablespoon garlic powder
- 1 tablespoon dried thyme
- 1 tablespoon olive oil

Instructions:

1. Preheat oven to 300°F (150°C).
2. Place ribs in a baking dish.
3. In a bowl, mix balsamic vinegar, honey, garlic powder, and thyme.
4. Brush the mixture over the ribs.
5. Cover with aluminum foil and bake in the preheated oven for about 2.5 hours, or until the meat is tender.
6. Remove foil, increase oven temperature to 400°F (200°C), and bake for an additional 30 minutes to caramelize the glaze.
7. Drizzle with olive oil and serve hot.

Nutritional Info per Serving:

- Calories: 680
- Protein: 58g
- Carbohydrates: 18g
- Fat: 40g
- Fiber: 0g
- Sugar: 16g

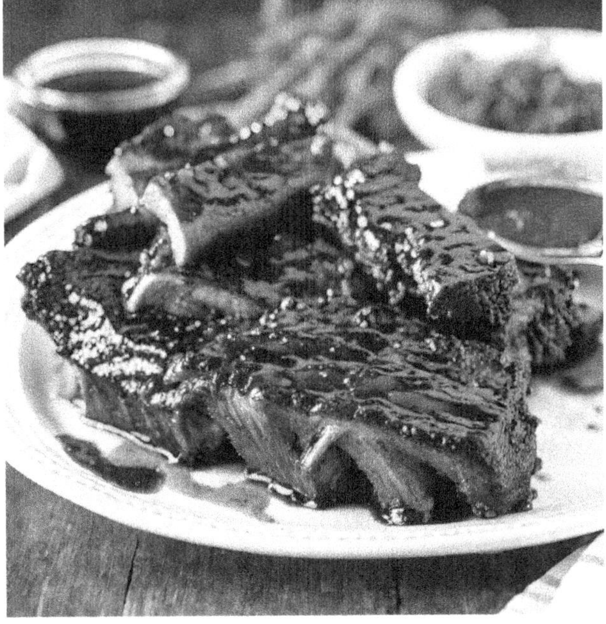

20. Roast Beef with Herbs

Servings: 6

Cooking Time: 1 hour 30 minutes

Ingredients:

- 3 pounds beef roast (such as sirloin tip)
- 1 tablespoon rosemary, minced
- 1 tablespoon thyme, minced
- 1 tablespoon sage, minced
- 1 tablespoon olive oil

Instructions:

1. Preheat oven to 375°F (190°C).
2. Rub the beef with olive oil and then coat with minced herbs.
3. Place in a roasting pan and roast in the preheated oven for about 1.5 hours, or until a thermometer inserted into the thickest part reaches 145°F (63°C) for medium rare.
4. Let rest for 15 minutes before slicing. Serve hot.

Nutritional Info per Serving:

- Calories: 380
- Protein: 50g
- Carbohydrates: 0g
- Fat: 20g
- Fiber: 0g
- Sugar: 0g

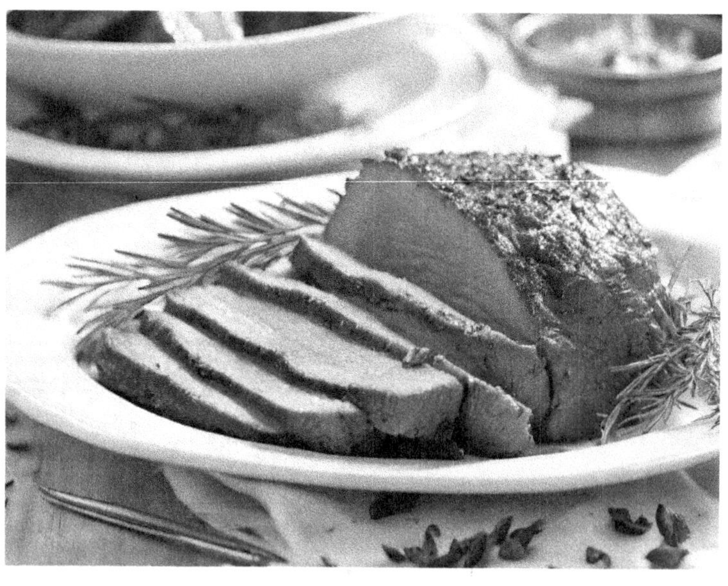

21. Beef and Spinach Meatballs

Servings: 4

Cooking Time: 30 minutes

Ingredients:

- 1 pound ground beef
- 2 cups spinach, finely chopped
- 1 onion, finely chopped
- 1 egg, beaten
- 1/4 cup almond flour
- 1 tablespoon olive oil

Instructions:

1. Preheat oven to 400°F (200°C).
2. In a bowl, combine ground beef, spinach, onion, egg, and almond flour.
3. Form the mixture into meatballs and place on a baking sheet.
4. Bake for 20-25 minutes, or until cooked through.
5. Drizzle with olive oil before serving.

Nutritional Info per Serving:

- Calories: 330
- Protein: 25g
- Carbohydrates: 5g
- Fat: 23g
- Fiber: 2g
- Sugar: 2g

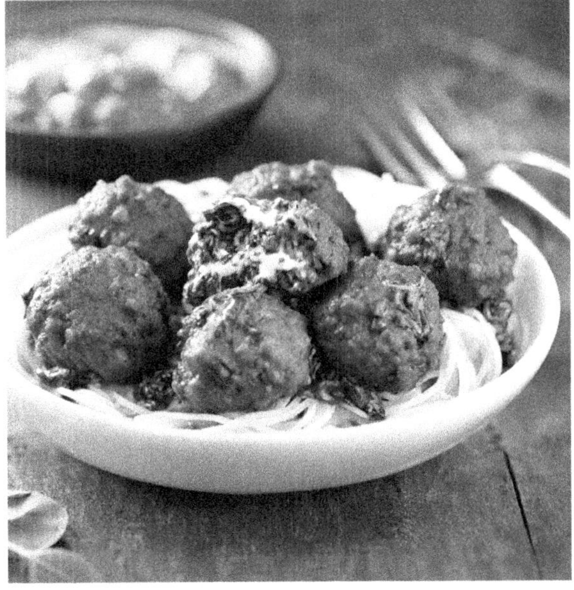

22. Grilled Ribeye Steak

Servings: 4
Cooking Time: 15 minutes
Ingredients:

- 4 ribeye steaks (about 12 oz each)
- 1 tablespoon garlic powder
- 1 tablespoon smoked paprika
- 1 tablespoon olive oil

Instructions:

1. Preheat grill to high heat.
2. Rub each steak with olive oil and then coat with garlic powder and smoked paprika.
3. Grill steaks for about 6-7 minutes per side for medium rare, or until desired doneness.
4. Let rest for 5 minutes before serving.

Nutritional Info per Serving:

- Calories: 560
- Protein: 45g
- Carbohydrates: 1g
- Fat: 42g
- Fiber: 0g
- Sugar: 0g

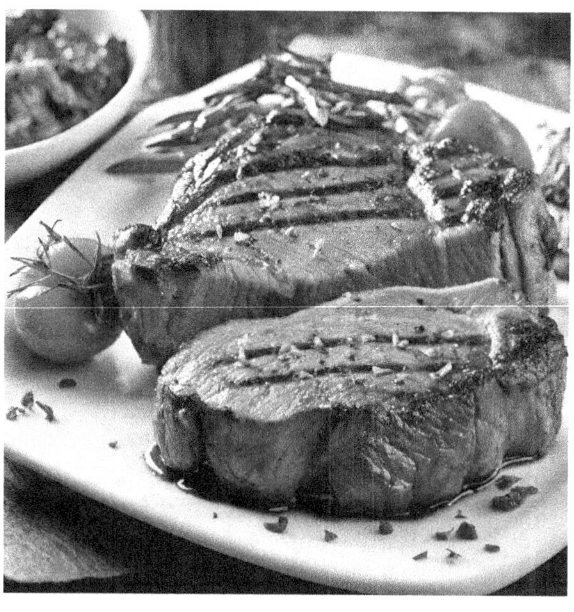

Vegetables

1. Roasted Pepper Salad with Garlic Dressing
Servings: 4
Cooking Time: 25 minutes
Ingredients:
- 4 bell peppers (red, yellow, and orange), sliced
- 2 cloves garlic, minced
- 1/4 cup olive oil
- 2 tablespoons red wine vinegar
- Fresh basil leaves, chopped

Instructions:
1. Preheat the oven to 425°F (220°C).
2. Place the bell peppers on a baking sheet and roast for 20 minutes or until charred and soft.
3. Whisk together olive oil, red wine vinegar, and minced garlic for the dressing.
4. Toss the roasted peppers in the garlic dressing.
5. Garnish with fresh basil before serving.

Nutritional Info per Serving:
- Calories: 180
- Protein: 1g
- Carbohydrates: 9g
- Fat: 15g
- Fiber: 3g
- Sugar: 6g

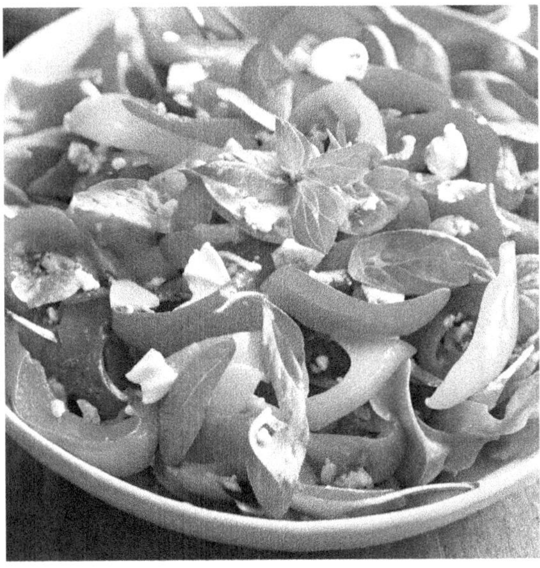

2. Coleslaw with Olive Oil and Vinegar

Servings: 4
Cooking Time: 15 minutes
Ingredients:

- 4 cups shredded cabbage
- 1 carrot, shredded
- 1/4 cup olive oil
- 1/4 cup apple cider vinegar
- 1 tablespoon honey
- Fresh dill, chopped

Instructions:

1. In a large bowl, combine shredded cabbage and carrot.
2. In a small bowl, whisk together olive oil, apple cider vinegar, and honey.
3. Pour the dressing over the cabbage and carrot mixture and toss well.
4. Garnish with chopped dill before serving.

Nutritional Info per Serving:

- Calories: 190
- Protein: 1g
- Carbohydrates: 10g
- Fat: 16g
- Fiber: 2g
- Sugar: 7g

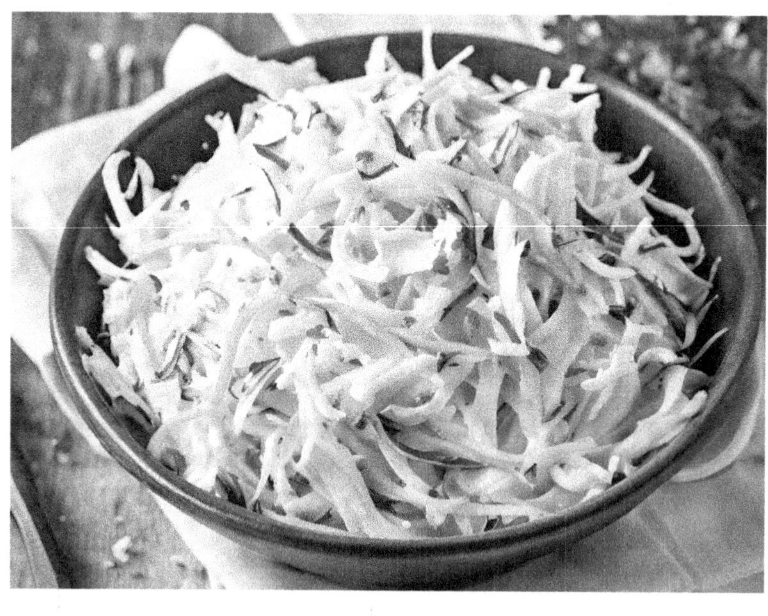

3. Endive and Apple Salad

Servings: 4
Cooking Time: 10 minutes
Ingredients:

- 4 endives, chopped
- 2 apples, thinly sliced
- 1/4 cup walnuts, chopped
- 2 tablespoons lemon juice
- 2 tablespoons olive oil
- Fresh mint, chopped

Instructions:

1. In a large salad bowl, combine chopped endives, sliced apples, and chopped walnuts.
2. Whisk together lemon juice and olive oil for the dressing.
3. Toss the salad with the dressing.
4. Garnish with chopped mint before serving.

Nutritional Info per Serving:

- Calories: 180
- Protein: 2g
- Carbohydrates: 14g
- Fat: 14g
- Fiber: 4g
- Sugar: 9g

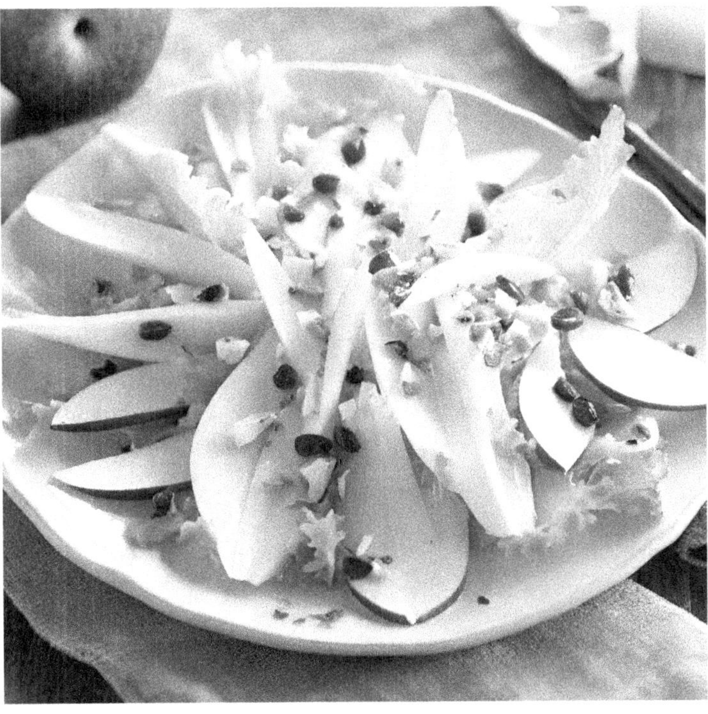

4. Fennel and Orange Salad

Servings: 4
Cooking Time: 15 minutes
Ingredients:

- 2 fennel bulbs, thinly sliced
- 2 oranges, peeled and segments
- 1/4 cup olive oil
- 2 tablespoons lemon juice
- Fresh parsley, chopped

Instructions:

1. In a salad bowl, combine thinly sliced fennel and orange segments.
2. Whisk together olive oil and lemon juice for the dressing.
3. Toss the salad with the dressing.
4. Garnish with chopped parsley before serving.

Nutritional Info per Serving:

- Calories: 190
- Protein: 2g
- Carbohydrates: 15g
- Fat: 14g
- Fiber: 4g
- Sugar: 10g

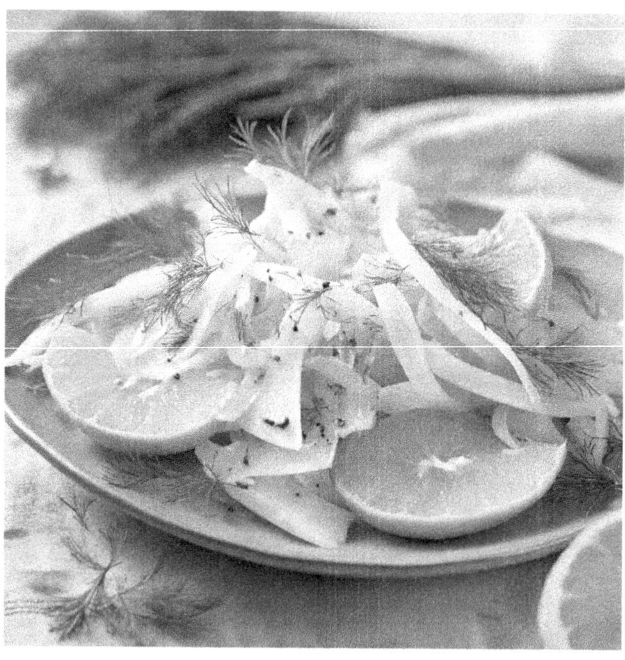

5. Shaved Brussels Sprouts with Lemon and Pecans

Servings: 4

Cooking Time: 20 minutes

Ingredients:

- 4 cups Brussels sprouts, trimmed and thinly sliced
- 1/4 cup pecans, chopped
- 2 tablespoons lemon juice
- 2 tablespoons olive oil
- Fresh thyme, chopped

Instructions:

1. In a large skillet, heat olive oil over medium heat.
2. Add the thinly sliced Brussels sprouts and sauté until tender and slightly caramelized, about 15 minutes.
3. Remove from heat and toss with lemon juice and chopped pecans.
4. Garnish with chopped thyme before serving.

Nutritional Info per Serving:

- Calories: 180
- Protein: 4g
- Carbohydrates: 10g
- Fat: 14g
- Fiber: 4g
- Sugar: 3g

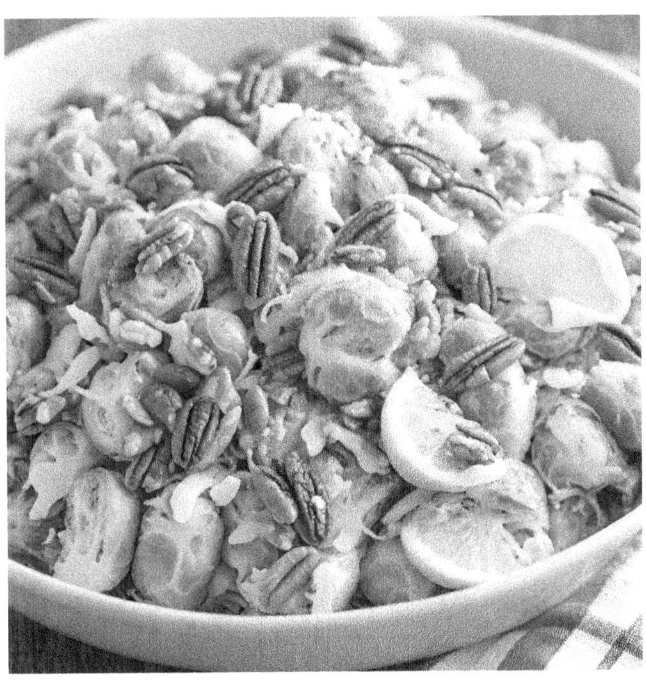

6. Spinach and Strawberry Salad

Servings: 4

Cooking Time: 10 minutes

Ingredients:

- 4 cups fresh spinach
- 1 cup strawberries, sliced
- 1/2 cup almonds, slivered
- 2 tablespoons balsamic vinegar
- 2 tablespoons olive oil
- Fresh basil, chopped

Instructions:

1. In a large salad bowl, combine fresh spinach, sliced strawberries, and slivered almonds.
2. Whisk together balsamic vinegar and olive oil for the dressing.
3. Toss the salad with the dressing.
4. Garnish with chopped basil before serving.

Nutritional Info per Serving:

- Calories: 200
- Protein: 4g
- Carbohydrates: 10g
- Fat: 16g
- Fiber: 3g
- Sugar: 5g

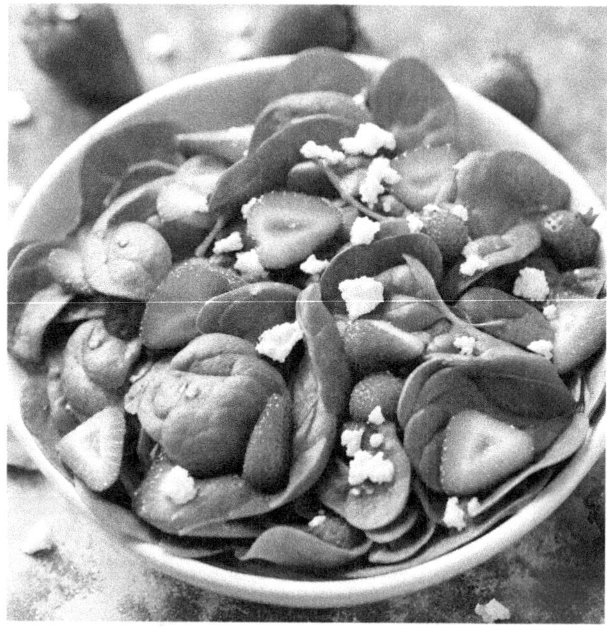

7. Stuffed Mushrooms with Spinach and Herbs

Servings: 4
Cooking Time: 25 minutes
Ingredients:

- 12 large mushrooms, stems removed
- 2 cups spinach, chopped
- 1 onion, finely chopped
- 2 cloves garlic, minced
- 1/4 cup almonds, finely chopped
- 2 tablespoons olive oil
- Fresh thyme, chopped

Instructions:

1. Preheat oven to 375°F (190°C).
2. Heat one tablespoon of olive oil in a skillet over medium heat. Sauté onion and garlic until translucent.
3. Add chopped spinach and cook until wilted. Remove from heat and mix in chopped almonds.
4. Stuff each mushroom cap with the spinach mixture.
5. Place stuffed mushrooms on a baking sheet, drizzle with the remaining olive oil.
6. Bake for 20 minutes, or until mushrooms are tender.
7. Garnish with chopped thyme before serving.

Nutritional Info per Serving:

- Calories: 150
- Protein: 5g
- Carbohydrates: 8g
- Fat: 12g
- Fiber: 3g
- Sugar: 3g

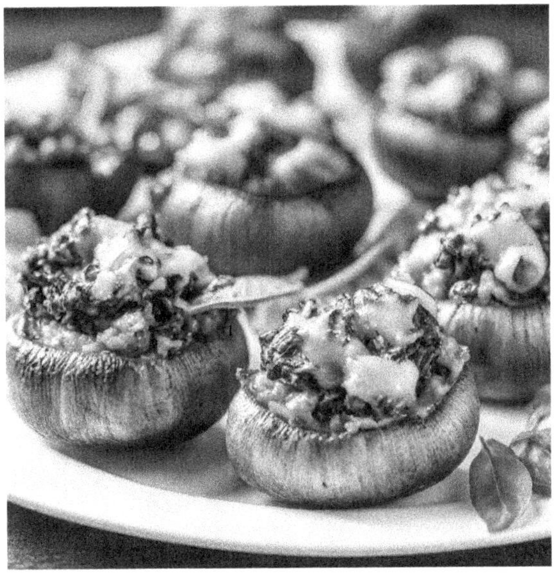

8. Roasted Turnips with Herbs
Servings: 4
Cooking Time: 35 minutes
Ingredients:
- 4 large turnips, peeled and cubed
- 2 tablespoons olive oil
- 1 tablespoon rosemary, chopped
- 1 tablespoon thyme, chopped

Instructions:
1. Preheat oven to 400°F (200°C).
2. Toss cubed turnips with olive oil, rosemary, and thyme.
3. Spread turnips on a baking sheet in a single layer.
4. Roast for 30 minutes, or until turnips are tender and golden.
5. Serve hot.

Nutritional Info per Serving:
- Calories: 120
- Protein: 2g
- Carbohydrates: 10g
- Fat: 8g
- Fiber: 3g
- Sugar: 5g

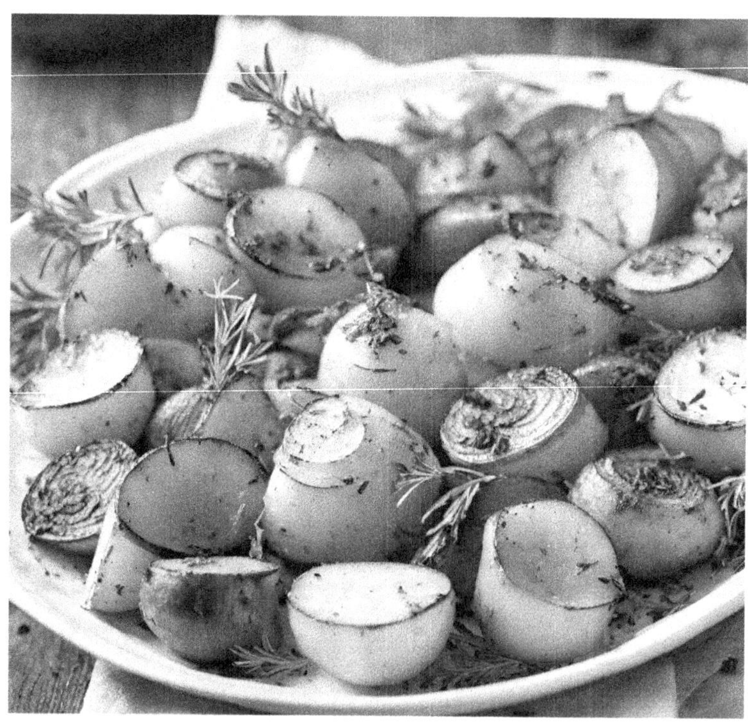

9. Roasted Garlic Eggplant

Servings: 4
Cooking Time: 40 minutes
Ingredients:

- 2 large eggplants, sliced into 1/2-inch thick rounds
- 4 cloves garlic, minced
- 1/4 cup olive oil
- Fresh parsley, chopped

Instructions:

1. Preheat oven to 400°F (200°C).
2. Arrange eggplant slices on a baking sheet.
3. Mix olive oil and minced garlic, and brush over eggplant slices.
4. Roast in the oven for 35 minutes, flipping halfway through, until eggplant is tender and golden brown.
5. Garnish with chopped parsley before serving.

Nutritional Info per Serving:

- Calories: 180
- Protein: 2g
- Carbohydrates: 15g
- Fat: 14g
- Fiber: 5g
- Sugar: 9g

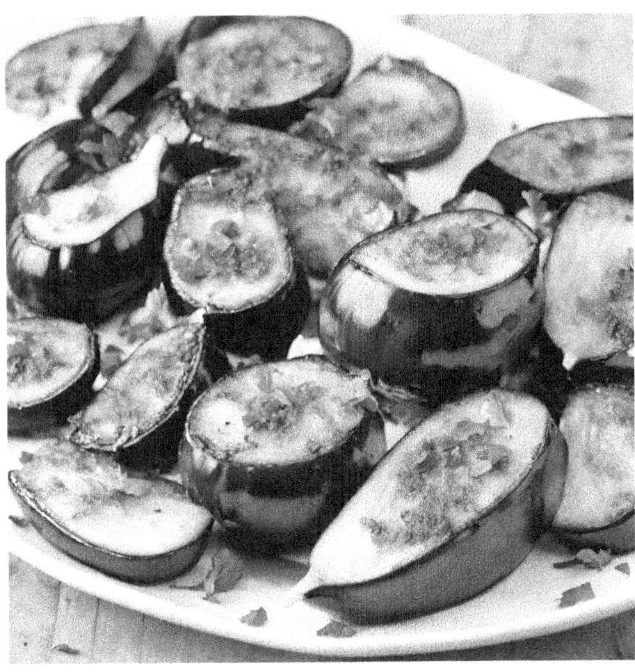

10. Herb Roasted Zucchini and Squash
Servings: 4
Cooking Time: 25 minutes
Ingredients:
- 2 zucchinis, sliced
- 2 yellow squashes, sliced
- 2 tablespoons olive oil
- 1 tablespoon rosemary, chopped
- 1 tablespoon thyme, chopped

Instructions:
1. Preheat oven to 425°F (220°C).
2. In a large bowl, toss zucchini and squash slices with olive oil, rosemary, and thyme.
3. Spread the vegetables in a single layer on a baking sheet.
4. Roast for 20 minutes, or until vegetables are tender and slightly browned.
5. Serve hot.

Nutritional Info per Serving:
- Calories: 110
- Protein: 2g
- Carbohydrates: 8g
- Fat: 8g
- Fiber: 2g
- Sugar: 4g

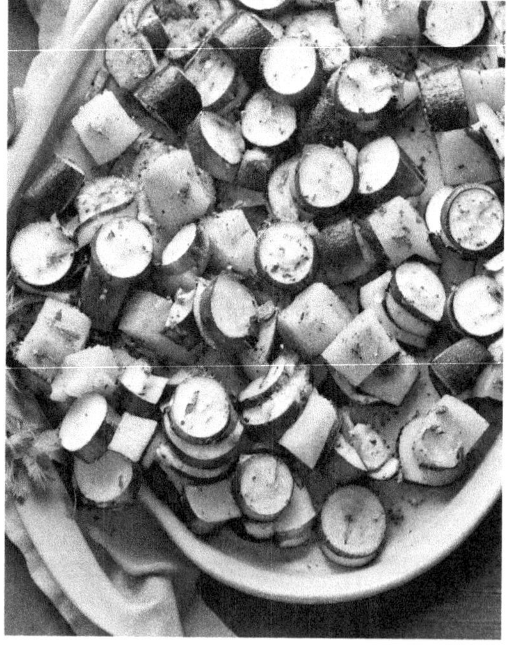

11. Broccoli and Almond Stir-Fry

Servings: 4
Cooking Time: 15 minutes
Ingredients:

- 4 cups broccoli florets
- 1/2 cup almonds, slivered
- 2 tablespoons sesame oil
- 2 cloves garlic, minced
- 2 tablespoons soy sauce (or tamari for gluten-free option)
- Fresh cilantro, chopped

Instructions:

1. Heat sesame oil in a large skillet over medium heat.
2. Add garlic and sauté for 1 minute until fragrant.
3. Add broccoli and stir-fry for about 5 minutes until it starts to become tender.
4. Add slivered almonds and soy sauce, and continue to stir-fry for another 5 minutes.
5. Garnish with chopped cilantro before serving.

Nutritional Info per Serving:

- Calories: 180
- Protein: 6g
- Carbohydrates: 10g
- Fat: 14g
- Fiber: 4g
- Sugar: 2g

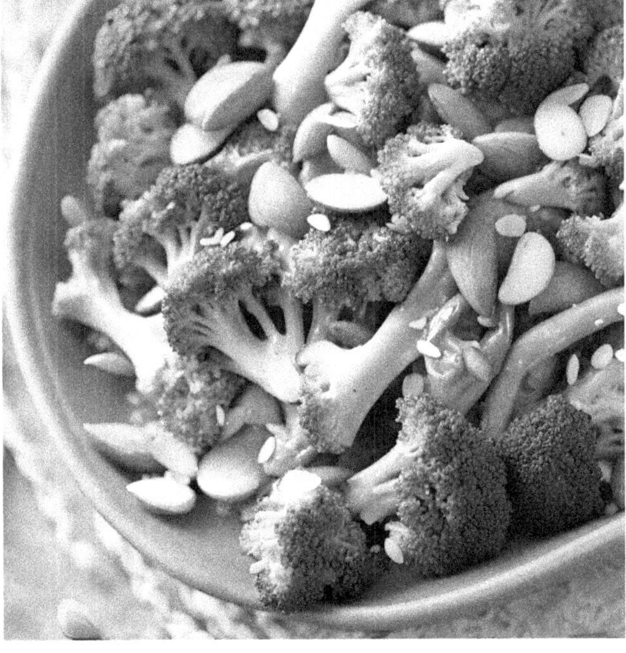

12. Baked Radishes with Olive Oil and Herbs

Servings: 4
Cooking Time: 25 minutes
Ingredients:

- 2 bunches radishes, halved
- 2 tablespoons olive oil
- 1 tablespoon rosemary, chopped
- 1 tablespoon thyme, chopped

Instructions:

1. Preheat oven to 400°F (200°C).
2. Toss radishes with olive oil, rosemary, and thyme.
3. Spread radishes on a baking sheet in a single layer.
4. Roast for 20 minutes, or until radishes are tender and slightly caramelized.
5. Serve hot.

Nutritional Info per Serving:

- Calories: 100
- Protein: 1g
- Carbohydrates: 4g
- Fat: 9g
- Fiber: 1g
- Sugar: 2g

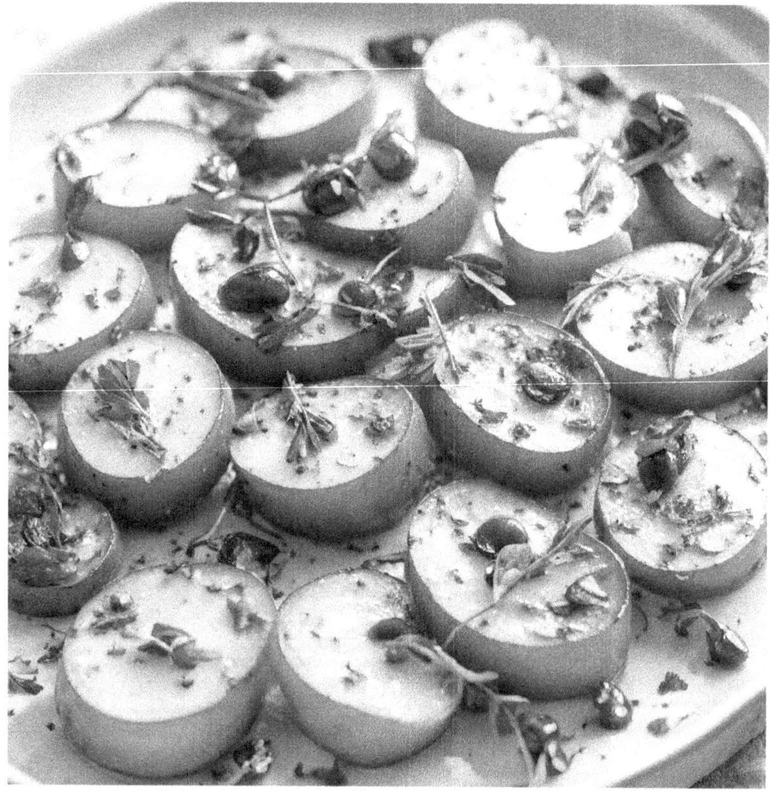

13. Cauliflower Rice Pilaf

Servings: 4
Cooking Time: 20 minutes
Ingredients:

- 1 head cauliflower, grated into rice-sized pieces
- 1 onion, finely chopped
- 1/4 cup carrots, finely diced
- 1/4 cup celery, finely diced
- 2 tablespoons olive oil
- Fresh parsley, chopped

Instructions:

1. Heat olive oil in a large skillet over medium heat.
2. Add onion, carrots, and celery, and sauté until soft.
3. Stir in grated cauliflower and continue to cook for about 10 minutes, stirring occasionally, until the cauliflower is tender.
4. Garnish with chopped parsley before serving.

Nutritional Info per Serving:

- Calories: 120
- Protein: 3g
- Carbohydrates: 12g
- Fat: 7g
- Fiber: 4g
- Sugar: 5g

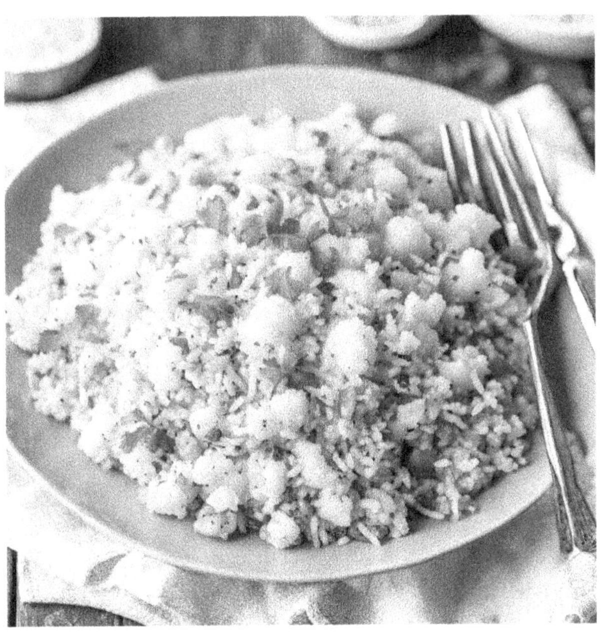

14. Grilled Artichokes with Lemon Aioli

Servings: 4

Cooking Time: 45 minutes

Ingredients:

- 4 artichokes, halved and cleaned
- 2 tablespoons olive oil
- 1/2 cup mayonnaise
- 1 lemon, juiced
- 1 garlic clove, minced

Instructions:

1. Preheat grill to medium-high heat.
2. Brush artichokes with olive oil.
3. Grill artichokes cut-side down for about 10 minutes, then flip and grill for another 10 minutes until tender.
4. Mix mayonnaise, lemon juice, and minced garlic to make aioli.
5. Serve grilled artichokes with lemon aioli.

Nutritional Info per Serving:

- Calories: 290
- Protein: 4g
- Carbohydrates: 14g
- Fat: 24g
- Fiber: 7g
- Sugar: 2g

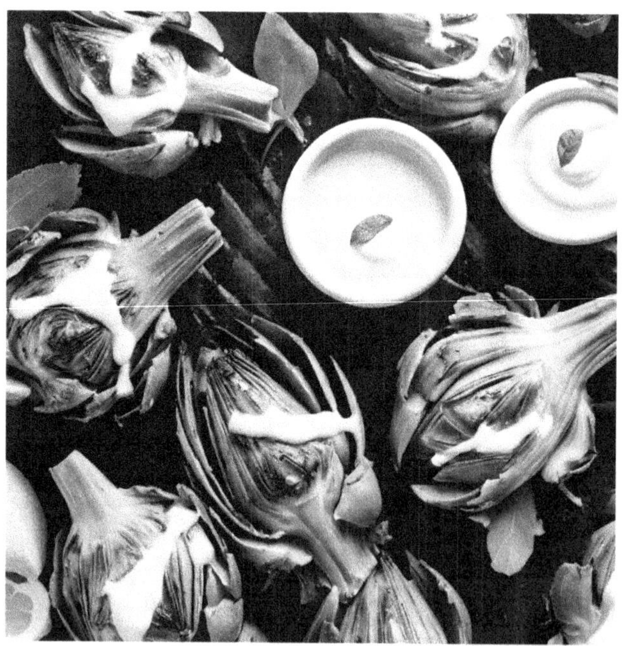

15. Zucchini Ribbons with Olive Oil and Lemon

Servings: 4
Cooking Time: 10 minutes
Ingredients:

- 4 zucchinis, thinly sliced into ribbons with a peeler or mandoline
- 2 tablespoons olive oil
- 1 lemon, juiced
- Fresh mint, chopped

Instructions:

1. In a large bowl, toss zucchini ribbons with olive oil and lemon juice.
2. Chill in the refrigerator for about 10 minutes to allow flavors to meld.
3. Garnish with chopped mint before serving.

Nutritional Info per Serving:

- Calories: 120
- Protein: 2g
- Carbohydrates: 6g
- Fat: 10g
- Fiber: 2g

Sugar: 3g

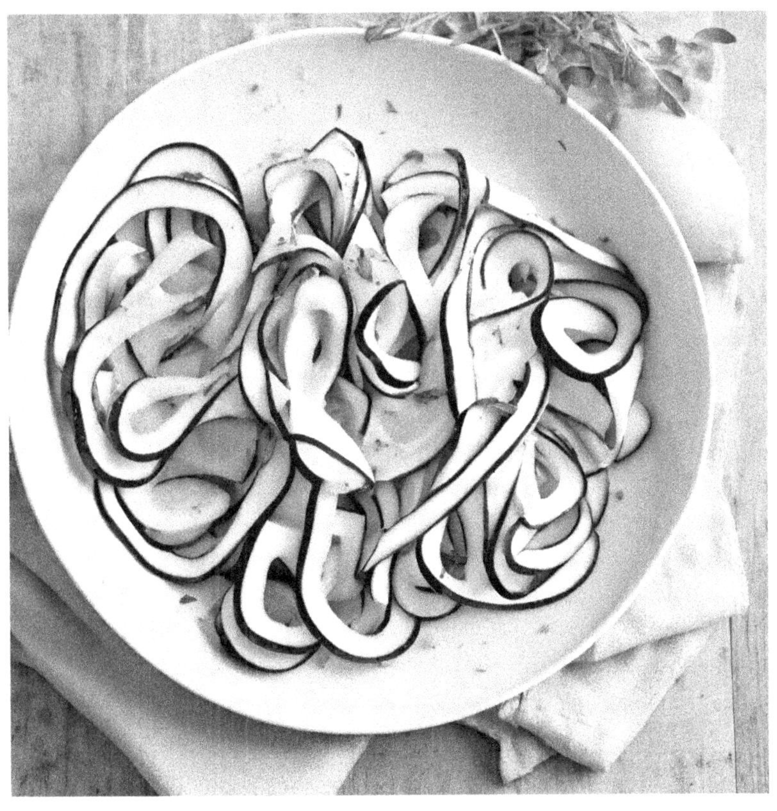

Fish & Seafood Recipes

1. Lemon Herb Grilled Salmon

Servings: 4
Cooking Time: 15 minutes
Ingredients:

- 4 salmon fillets
- 2 tablespoons olive oil
- 2 tablespoons lemon juice
- 2 cloves garlic, minced
- 1 tablespoon fresh dill, chopped
- 1 tablespoon fresh parsley, chopped

Instructions:

1. Preheat grill to medium-high heat.
2. In a small bowl, mix olive oil, lemon juice, minced garlic, dill, and parsley to create a marinade.
3. Place salmon fillets in a shallow dish and pour marinade over them. Let marinate for 10 minutes.
4. Grill salmon for about 6-8 minutes per side, or until cooked through and flaky.
5. Serve hot.

Nutritional Info per Serving:

- Calories: 320
- Protein: 34g
- Carbohydrates: 2g
- Fat: 20g
- Fiber: 0g
- Sugar: 0g

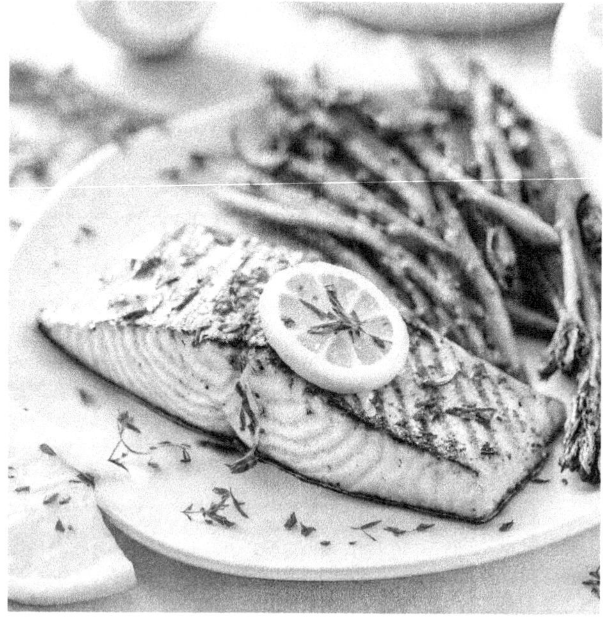

2. Garlic Butter Baked Cod

Servings: 4
Cooking Time: 20 minutes
Ingredients:

- 4 cod fillets
- 4 tablespoons butter, melted
- 4 cloves garlic, minced
- 1 tablespoon lemon juice
- 1 tablespoon fresh parsley, chopped

Instructions:

1. Preheat oven to 400°F (200°C).
2. Place cod fillets in a baking dish.
3. In a small bowl, mix melted butter, minced garlic, lemon juice, and chopped parsley.
4. Pour the butter mixture over the cod fillets.
5. Bake for 15-20 minutes, or until fish is cooked through and flakes easily with a fork.
6. Serve hot.

Nutritional Info per Serving:

- Calories: 230
- Protein: 27g
- Carbohydrates: 2g
- Fat: 13g
- Fiber: 0g
- Sugar: 0g

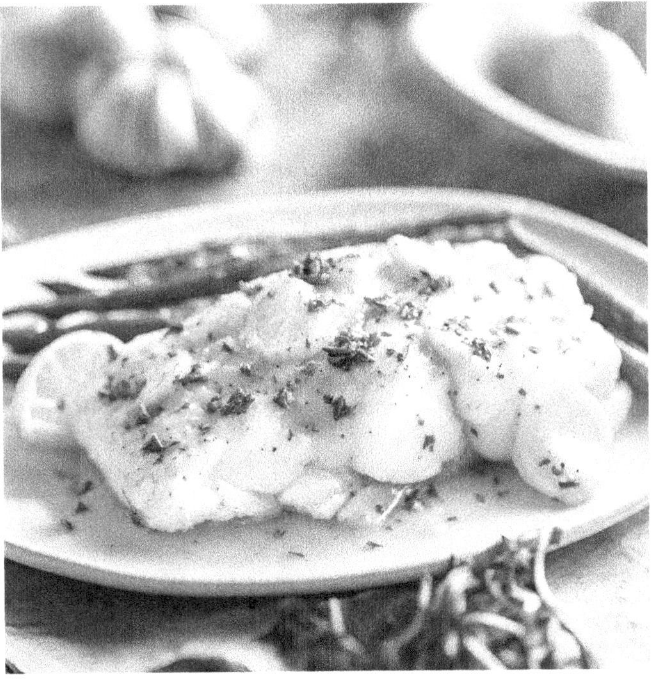

3. Spicy Grilled Mackerel

Servings: 4
Cooking Time: 10 minutes
Ingredients:

- 4 mackerel fillets
- 2 tablespoons olive oil
- 1 tablespoon paprika
- 1 teaspoon cayenne pepper
- 1 teaspoon garlic powder
- 1 teaspoon onion powder
- 1 teaspoon dried thyme

Instructions:

1. Preheat grill to medium-high heat.
2. In a small bowl, mix olive oil, paprika, cayenne pepper, garlic powder, onion powder, and dried thyme to create a spice rub.
3. Rub spice mixture evenly over both sides of the mackerel fillets.
4. Grill mackerel for about 4-5 minutes per side, or until cooked through.
5. Serve hot.

Nutritional Info per Serving:

- Calories: 280
- Protein: 25g
- Carbohydrates: 2g
- Fat: 19g
- Fiber: 1g
- Sugar: 0g

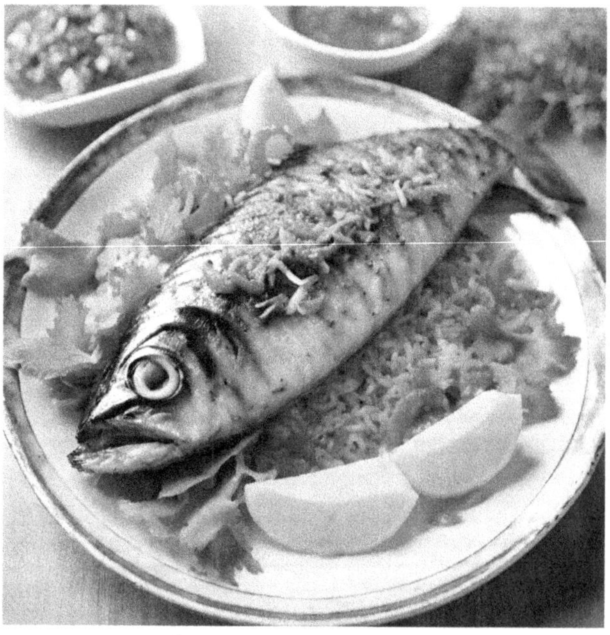

4. Pesto-Rubbed Tuna Steaks

Servings: 4
Cooking Time: 10 minutes
Ingredients:

- 4 tuna steaks
- 4 tablespoons pesto sauce
- 2 tablespoons olive oil
- Salt and pepper to taste

Instructions:

1. Preheat grill to high heat.
2. Brush both sides of tuna steaks with olive oil and season with salt and pepper.
3. Spread pesto sauce evenly over both sides of the tuna steaks.
4. Grill tuna steaks for about 2-3 minutes per side for medium-rare, or until desired doneness.
5. Serve hot.

Nutritional Info per Serving:

- Calories: 320
- Protein: 34g
- Carbohydrates: 2g
- Fat: 20g
- Fiber: 0g
- Sugar: 0g

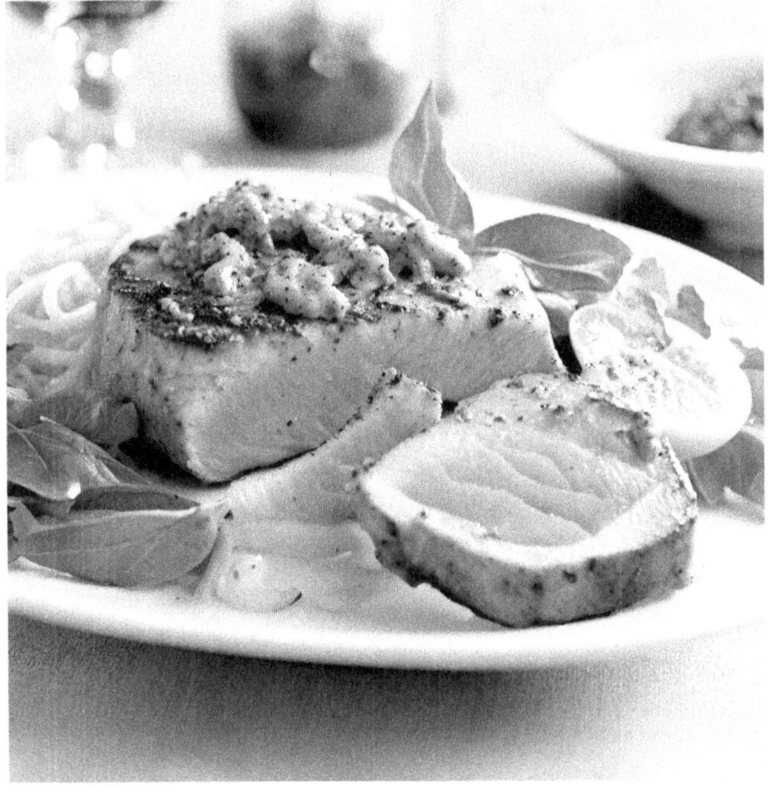

5. Baked Trout with Fennel

Servings: 4
Cooking Time: 25 minutes
Ingredients:

- 4 trout fillets
- 2 tablespoons olive oil
- 1 lemon, sliced
- 1 fennel bulb, thinly sliced
- Salt and pepper to taste

Instructions:

1. Preheat oven to 375°F (190°C).
2. Place trout fillets on a baking sheet lined with parchment paper.
3. Drizzle olive oil over the trout fillets and season with salt and pepper.
4. Arrange lemon slices and thinly sliced fennel on top of the trout fillets.
5. Bake for 20-25 minutes, or until fish is cooked through and flakes easily with a fork.
6. Serve hot.

Nutritional Info per Serving:

- Calories: 240
- Protein: 24g
- Carbohydrates: 6g
- Fat: 14g
- Fiber: 2G
- Sugar: 3g

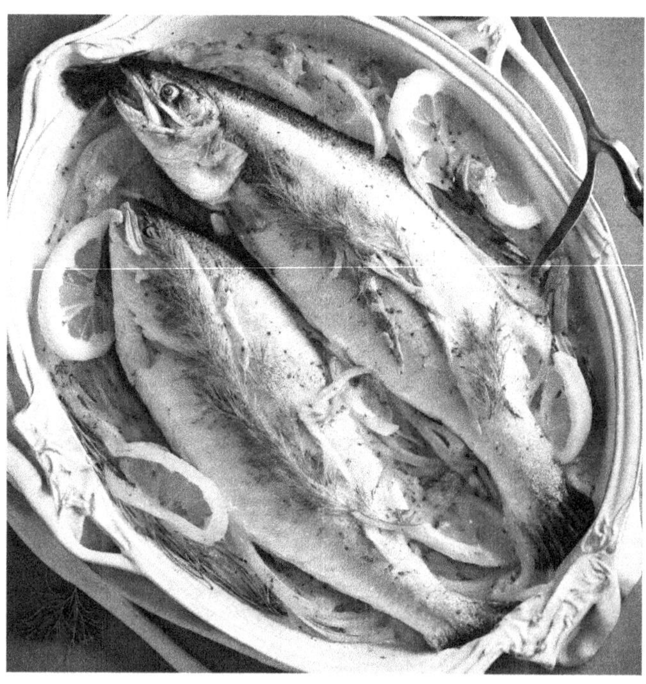

6. Herbed Halibut in Foil

Servings: 4
Cooking Time: 20 minutes
Ingredients:
- 4 halibut fillets
- 2 tablespoons olive oil
- 2 cloves garlic, minced
- 1 tablespoon fresh parsley, chopped
- 1 tablespoon fresh dill, chopped
- 1 tablespoon lemon juice
- Salt and pepper to taste

Instructions:
1. Preheat oven to 375°F (190°C).
2. Place each halibut fillet on a piece of aluminum foil large enough to wrap it.
3. In a small bowl, mix olive oil, minced garlic, chopped parsley, chopped dill, lemon juice, salt, and pepper.
4. Brush each halibut fillet with the herb mixture, then fold the foil over to create a packet.
5. Place the foil packets on a baking sheet and bake for 15-20 minutes, or until fish is cooked through and flakes easily with a fork.
6. Serve hot, directly from the foil packets.

Nutritional Info per Serving:
- Calories: 220
- Protein: 30g
- Carbohydrates: 1g
- Fat: 10g
- Fiber: 0g
- Sugar: 0g

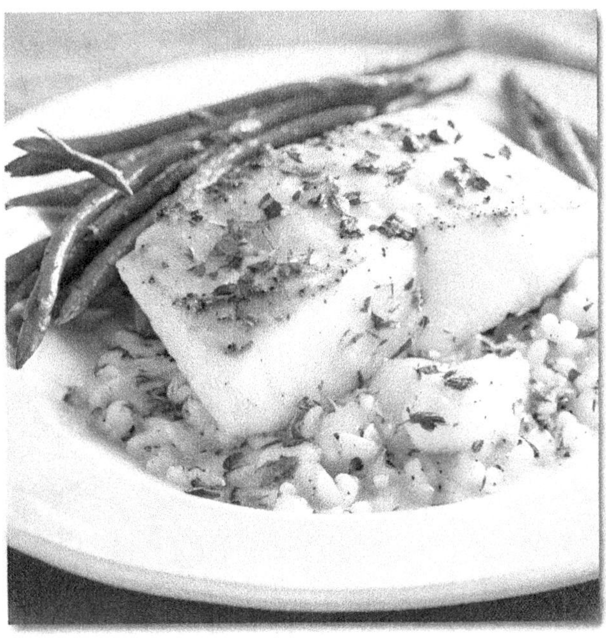

7. Grilled Catfish with Cajun Spices

Servings: 4
Cooking Time: 15 minutes
Ingredients:

- 4 catfish fillets
- 2 tablespoons olive oil
- 1 tablespoon paprika
- 1 teaspoon garlic powder
- 1 teaspoon onion powder
- 1 teaspoon dried thyme
- 1/2 teaspoon cayenne pepper
- 1/2 teaspoon black pepper
- 1/2 teaspoon salt

Instructions:

1. Preheat grill to medium-high heat.
2. In a small bowl, mix olive oil, paprika, garlic powder, onion powder, dried thyme, cayenne pepper, black pepper, and salt to create a spice rub.
3. Rub spice mixture evenly over both sides of the catfish fillets.
4. Grill catfish for about 5-7 minutes per side, or until fish is cooked through and flakes easily with a fork.
5. Serve hot.

Nutritional Info per Serving:

- Calories: 220
- Protein: 30g
- Carbohydrates: 2g
- Fat: 10g
- Fiber: 1g
- Sugar: 0g

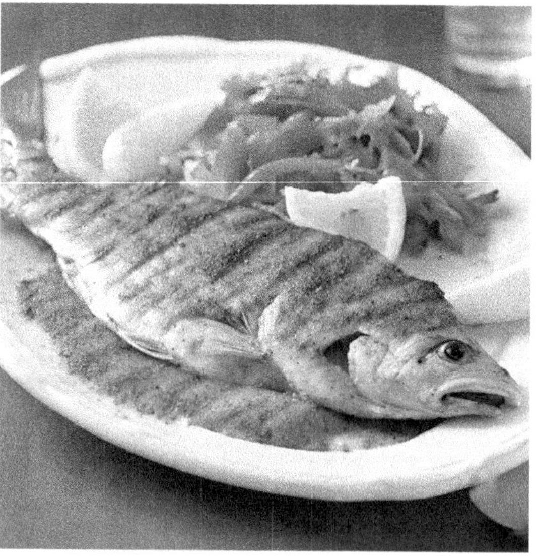

8. Spicy Shrimp Soup

Servings: 4
Cooking Time: 25 minutes
Ingredients:

- 1 pound shrimp, peeled and deveined
- 1 onion, diced
- 2 cloves garlic, minced
- 1 bell pepper, diced
- 1 jalapeño pepper, diced
- 1 can (14 oz) diced tomatoes
- 4 cups vegetable or chicken broth
- 1 teaspoon paprika
- 1/2 teaspoon cayenne pepper
- Salt and pepper to taste
- Fresh cilantro, chopped (for garnish)

Instructions:

1. In a large pot, heat olive oil over medium heat. Add diced onion, minced garlic, diced bell pepper, and diced jalapeño pepper. Sauté until vegetables are softened.
2. Add diced tomatoes (with juices) and broth to the pot. Bring to a simmer.
3. Stir in paprika, cayenne pepper, salt, and pepper. Simmer for 10-15 minutes to allow flavors to meld.
4. Add shrimp to the pot and cook for 5-7 minutes, or until shrimp are pink and cooked through.
5. Adjust seasoning if needed. Serve hot, garnished with chopped cilantro.

Nutritional Info per Serving:

- Calories: 180
- Protein: 25g
- Carbohydrates: 10g
- Fat: 4g
- Fiber: 3g
- Sugar: 5g

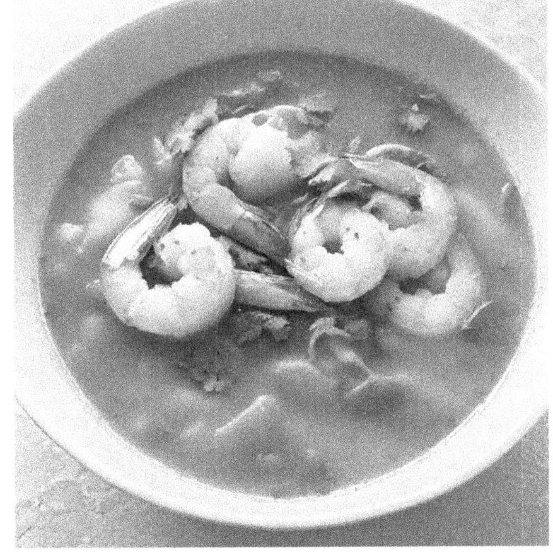

9. Creamy Salmon Soup

Servings: 4

Cooking Time: 25 minutes

Ingredients:

- 1 pound salmon fillets, skin removed and cut into chunks
- 1 onion, diced
- 2 cloves garlic, minced
- 2 cups chicken or vegetable broth
- 1 cup coconut milk
- 1 cup spinach leaves
- 2 tablespoons olive oil
- 1 tablespoon fresh dill, chopped
- 1 tablespoon lemon juice

Instructions:

1. In a large pot, heat olive oil over medium heat. Add diced onion and minced garlic. Sauté until softened.
2. Add salmon chunks to the pot and cook until lightly browned on the outside.
3. Pour in chicken or vegetable broth and bring to a simmer. Let simmer for 10 minutes.
4. Stir in coconut milk, spinach leaves, chopped dill, and lemon juice. Simmer for another 5 minutes.
5. Serve hot.

Nutritional Info per Serving:

- Calories: 320
- Protein: 22g
- Carbohydrates: 8g
- Fat: 24g
- Fiber: 2g
- Sugar: 3g

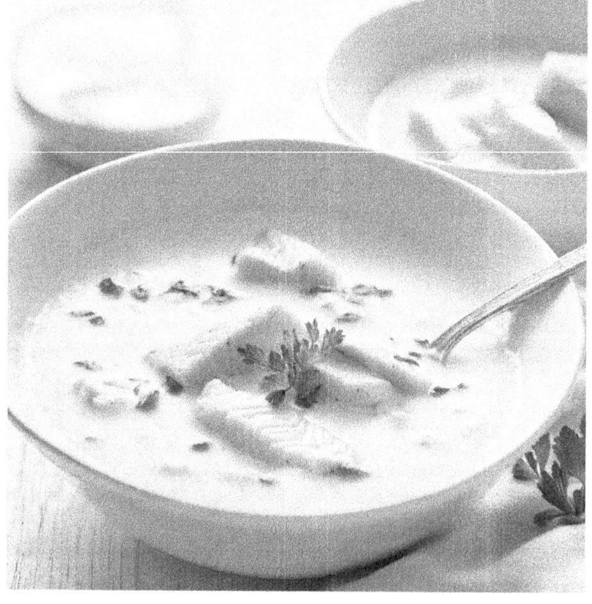

10. Clam and Vegetable Soup

Servings: 4
Cooking Time: 30 minutes
Ingredients:

- 2 cans (10 oz each) whole baby clams, drained
- 1 onion, diced
- 2 cloves garlic, minced
- 2 carrots, diced
- 2 celery stalks, diced
- 4 cups vegetable broth
- 1 cup diced tomatoes
- 1 teaspoon dried thyme
- Salt and pepper to taste
- Fresh parsley, chopped (for garnish)

Instructions:

1. In a large pot, heat olive oil over medium heat. Add diced onion and minced garlic. Sauté until softened.
2. Add diced carrots and celery to the pot. Cook for 5 minutes, until vegetables start to soften.
3. Pour in vegetable broth and bring to a simmer. Add diced tomatoes, dried thyme, salt, and pepper. Simmer for 15 minutes.
4. Stir in drained baby clams and simmer for another 5 minutes.
5. Serve hot, garnished with chopped parsley.

Nutritional Info per Serving:

- Calories: 180
- Protein: 14g
- Carbohydrates: 20g
- Fat: 4g
- Fiber: 4g
- Sugar: 6g

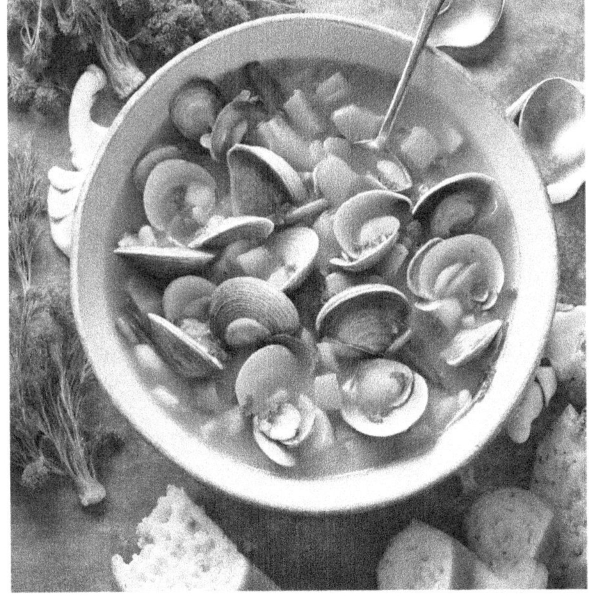

11. Cioppino

Servings: 4
Cooking Time: 45 minutes
Ingredients:

- 1 pound mixed seafood (such as shrimp, scallops, mussels, and white fish)
- 1 onion, diced
- 2 cloves garlic, minced
- 1 bell pepper, diced
- 1 can (14 oz) diced tomatoes
- 2 cups vegetable or fish broth
- 1/2 cup dry white wine (optional)
- 1 teaspoon dried oregano
- 1 teaspoon dried basil
- Salt and pepper to taste
- Fresh basil, chopped (for garnish)

Instructions:

1. In a large pot, heat olive oil over medium heat. Add diced onion, minced garlic, and diced bell pepper. Sauté until softened.
2. Add diced tomatoes, vegetable or fish broth, dry white wine (if using), dried oregano, dried basil, salt, and pepper. Bring to a simmer.
3. Simmer for 30 minutes to allow flavors to meld.
4. Add mixed seafood to the pot and cook for 5-10 minutes, or until seafood is cooked through.
5. Serve hot, garnished with chopped fresh basil.

Nutritional Info per Serving:

- Calories: 250
- Protein: 25g
- Carbohydrates: 14g
- Fat: 8g
- Fiber: 3g
- Sugar: 6g

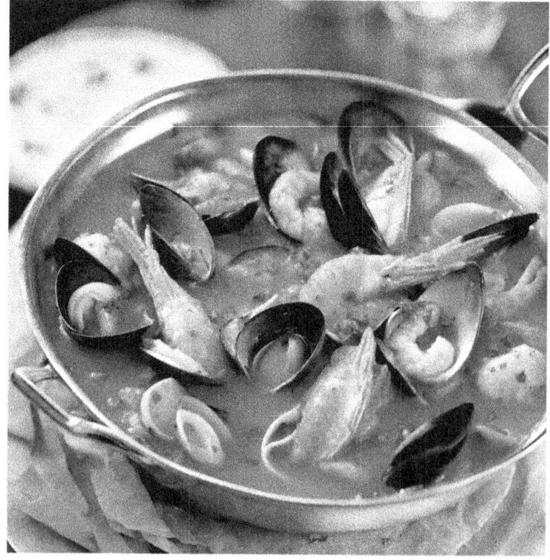

12. Cilantro Lime Shrimp Stew

Servings: 4
Cooking Time: 25 minutes
Ingredients:

- 1 pound shrimp, peeled and deveined
- 1 onion, diced
- 2 cloves garlic, minced
- 1 bell pepper, diced
- 1 can (14 oz) diced tomatoes
- 2 cups vegetable or chicken broth
- 1/4 cup chopped cilantro
- 2 tablespoons lime juice
- Salt and pepper to taste
- Avocado slices (for garnish)

Instructions:

1. In a large pot, heat olive oil over medium heat. Add diced onion, minced garlic, and diced bell pepper. Sauté until softened.
2. Add diced tomatoes, vegetable or chicken broth, chopped cilantro, lime juice, salt, and pepper. Bring to a simmer.
3. Simmer for 15 minutes to allow flavors to meld.
4. Add shrimp to the pot and cook for 5-7 minutes, or until shrimp are pink and cooked through.
5. Serve hot, garnished with avocado slices.

Nutritional Info per Serving:

- Calories: 200
- Protein: 25g
- Carbohydrates: 10g
- Fat: 5g
- Fiber: 3g
- Sugar: 5g

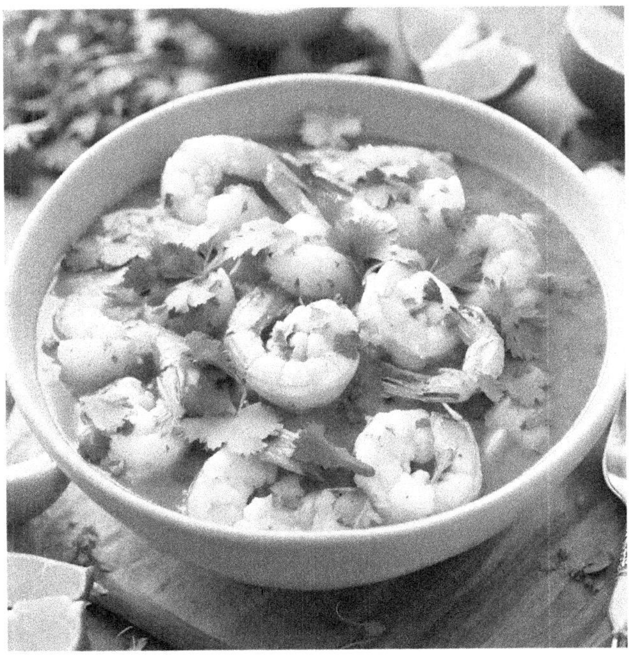

13. Smoked Salmon Salad

Servings: 4
Preparation Time: 15 minutes
Ingredients:

- 8 oz smoked salmon, thinly sliced
- 4 cups mixed salad greens
- 1 cucumber, sliced
- 1/2 red onion, thinly sliced
- 1/4 cup cherry tomatoes, halved
- 1/4 cup Kalamata olives, pitted
- 2 tablespoons capers
- 2 tablespoons olive oil
- 1 tablespoon lemon juice
- 1 teaspoon Dijon mustard
- Salt and pepper to taste

Instructions:

1. In a large salad bowl, combine the mixed greens, cucumber slices, red onion slices, cherry tomatoes, Kalamata olives, and capers.
2. In a small bowl, whisk together the olive oil, lemon juice, Dijon mustard, salt, and pepper to make the dressing.
3. Drizzle the dressing over the salad and toss to coat evenly.
4. Arrange the smoked salmon slices on top of the salad.
5. Serve immediately.

Nutritional Info per Serving:

- Calories: 220
- Protein: 20g
- Carbohydrates: 6g
- Fat: 14g
- Fiber: 2g
- Sugar: 2g

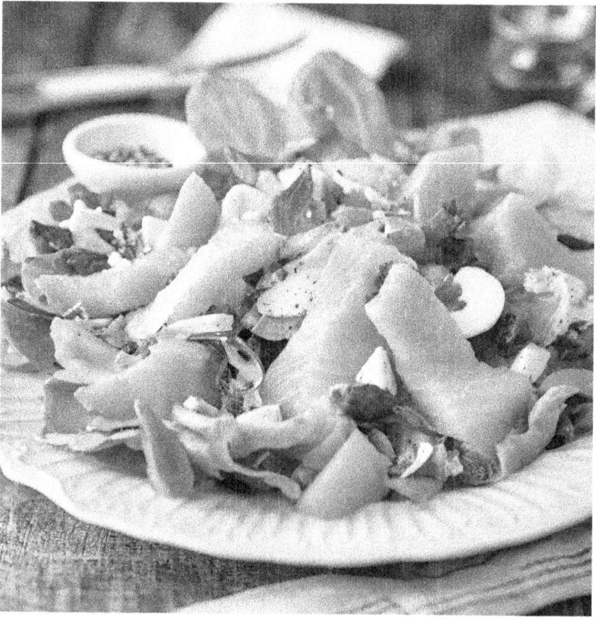

14. Tuna and Avocado Ceviche

Servings: 4
Preparation Time: 20 minutes (plus chilling time)
Ingredients:

- 1 pound sushi-grade tuna, diced
- 2 ripe avocados, diced
- 1/2 red onion, finely chopped
- 1 jalapeño pepper, seeded and minced
- 1/4 cup chopped fresh cilantro
- 1/4 cup lime juice
- 2 tablespoons orange juice
- Salt and pepper to taste
- Tortilla chips or lettuce leaves, for serving

Instructions:

1. In a large bowl, combine the diced tuna, diced avocado, chopped red onion, minced jalapeño pepper, and chopped cilantro.
2. In a small bowl, whisk together the lime juice, orange juice, salt, and pepper to make the marinade.
3. Pour the marinade over the tuna and avocado mixture, and gently toss to coat.
4. Cover the bowl and refrigerate for at least 30 minutes to allow the flavors to meld.
5. Serve the ceviche chilled, with tortilla chips or lettuce leaves for scooping.

Nutritional Info per Serving:

- Calories: 280
- Protein: 30g
- Carbohydrates: 10g
- Fat: 14g
- Fiber: 6g
- Sugar: 2g

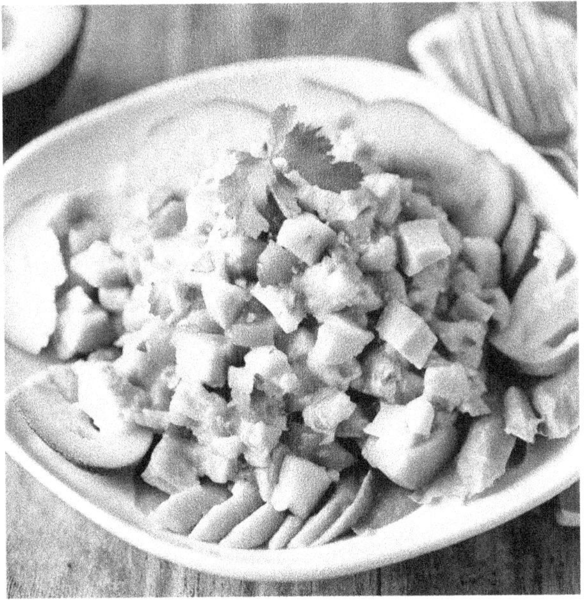

15. Shrimp and Cucumber Noodle Salad

Servings: 4

Preparation Time: 20 minutes

Ingredients:

- 1 pound cooked shrimp, peeled and deveined
- 2 large cucumbers, spiralized or julienned
- 1/2 red bell pepper, thinly sliced
- 1/4 cup chopped fresh cilantro
- 2 tablespoons sesame seeds
- 2 tablespoons rice vinegar
- 1 tablespoon soy sauce (or tamari for gluten-free)
- 1 tablespoon sesame oil
- 1 teaspoon honey
- 1 teaspoon grated ginger
- Salt and pepper to taste

Instructions:

1. In a large bowl, combine the cooked shrimp, cucumber noodles, sliced red bell pepper, chopped cilantro, and sesame seeds.
2. In a small bowl, whisk together the rice vinegar, soy sauce, sesame oil, honey, grated ginger, salt, and pepper to make the dressing.
3. Pour the dressing over the shrimp and cucumber noodle mixture, and toss to coat evenly.
4. Serve immediately, or refrigerate until ready to serve.

Nutritional Info per Serving:

- Calories: 220
- Protein: 25g
- Carbohydrates: 10g
- Fat: 8g
- Fiber: 2g
- Sugar: 5g

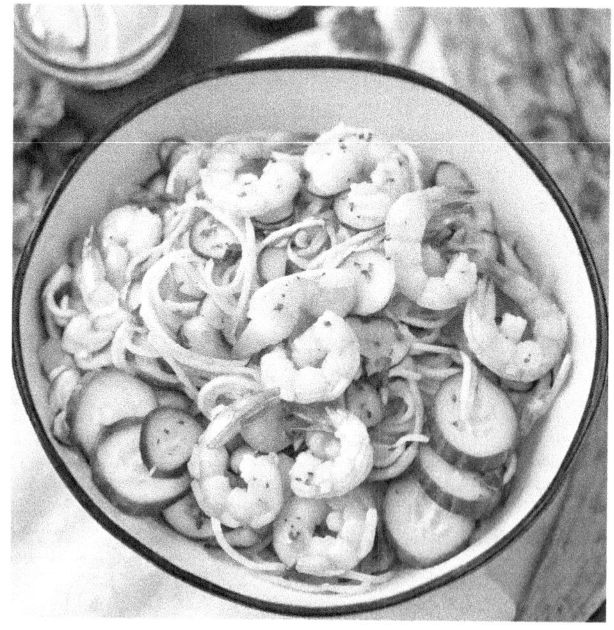

16. Octopus and Potato Salad

Servings: 4
Preparation Time: 30 minutes
Ingredients:

- 1 pound cooked octopus, diced
- 2 large potatoes, boiled and diced
- 1/2 red onion, thinly sliced
- 1/4 cup chopped fresh parsley
- 2 tablespoons olive oil
- 2 tablespoons lemon juice
- Salt and pepper to taste

Instructions:

1. In a large bowl, combine the diced octopus, diced potatoes, sliced red onion, and chopped parsley.
2. In a small bowl, whisk together the olive oil, lemon juice, salt, and pepper to make the dressing.
3. Pour the dressing over the octopus and potato mixture, and toss to coat evenly.
4. Serve the salad chilled or at room temperature.

Nutritional Info per Serving:

- Calories: 240
- Protein: 20g
- Carbohydrates: 20g
- Fat: 8g
- Fiber: 3g
- Sugar: 2g

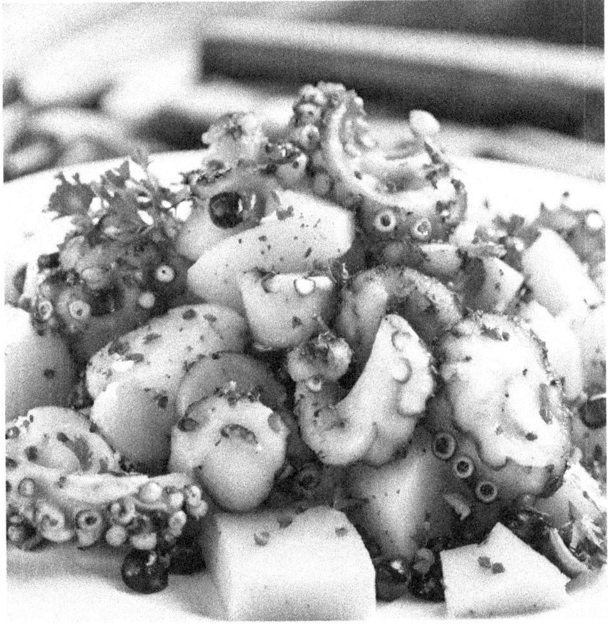

17. Crab and Avocado Stack

Servings: 4

Preparation Time: 15 minutes

Ingredients:

- 1 pound lump crab meat
- 2 ripe avocados, diced
- 1/4 cup diced red bell pepper
- 2 tablespoons chopped fresh cilantro
- 1 tablespoon lime juice
- 1 tablespoon olive oil
- Salt and pepper to taste
- Tortilla chips or lettuce leaves, for serving

Instructions:

1. In a bowl, gently mix together the lump crab meat, diced avocado, diced red bell pepper, chopped cilantro, lime juice, olive oil, salt, and pepper.
2. Divide the mixture into four portions.
3. Using a ring mold or a clean, empty can, place one portion of the crab and avocado mixture into the mold and press down gently to compact.
4. Carefully remove the mold to reveal a crab and avocado stack.
5. Repeat with the remaining portions of the mixture to create four stacks.
6. Serve the crab and avocado stacks with tortilla chips or lettuce leaves for scooping.

Nutritional Info per Serving:

- Calories: 240
- Protein: 20g
- Carbohydrates: 8g
- Fat: 14g
- Fiber: 6g
- Sugar: 2g

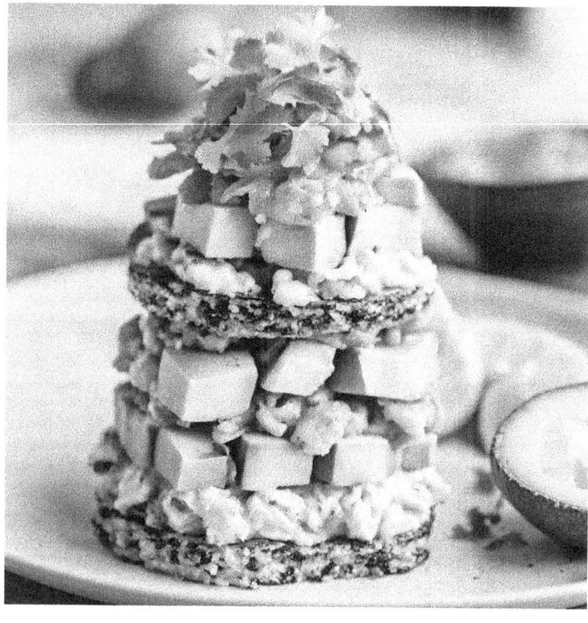

18. Pan-Seared Scallops with Lemon Butter

Servings: 4

Cooking Time: 10 minutes

Ingredients:
- 1 pound fresh scallops
- 2 tablespoons olive oil
- 2 tablespoons butter
- 2 cloves garlic, minced
- 2 tablespoons lemon juice
- 1 tablespoon chopped fresh parsley
- Salt and pepper to taste

Instructions:
1. Pat the scallops dry with paper towels and season with salt and pepper.
2. Heat olive oil in a large skillet over medium-high heat.
3. Add the scallops to the skillet and cook for 2-3 minutes on each side, or until golden brown and cooked through.
4. Remove the scallops from the skillet and set aside.
5. In the same skillet, melt the butter over medium heat. Add minced garlic and cook for 1 minute, until fragrant.
6. Stir in lemon juice and chopped parsley, then return the scallops to the skillet. Cook for another minute, spooning the lemon butter sauce over the scallops.
7. Serve hot.

Nutritional Info per Serving:
- Calories: 220
- Protein: 25g
- Carbohydrates: 2g
- Fat: 12g
- Fiber: 0g
- Sugar: 0g

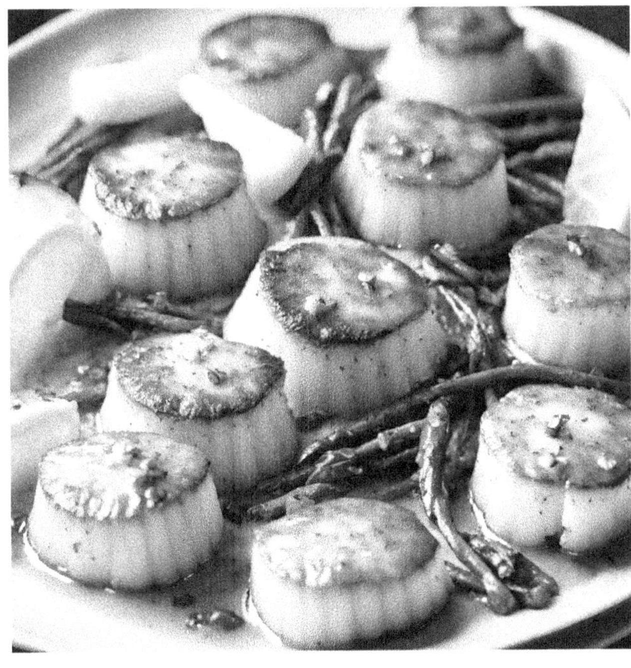

19. Stir-Fried Shrimp and Broccoli

Servings: 4
Cooking Time: 15 minutes
Ingredients:

- 1 pound shrimp, peeled and deveined
- 2 cups broccoli florets
- 1 bell pepper, sliced
- 2 cloves garlic, minced
- 2 tablespoons olive oil
- 2 tablespoons soy sauce (or tamari for gluten-free)
- 1 tablespoon oyster sauce
- 1 teaspoon sesame oil
- 1 teaspoon grated ginger
- Sesame seeds for garnish (optional)

Instructions:

1. Heat olive oil in a large skillet or wok over medium-high heat.
2. Add minced garlic and grated ginger to the skillet and cook for 1 minute, until fragrant.
3. Add shrimp to the skillet and stir-fry for 2-3 minutes, until pink and cooked through. Remove shrimp from the skillet and set aside.
4. In the same skillet, add broccoli florets and sliced bell pepper. Stir-fry for 3-4 minutes, until vegetables are tender-crisp.
5. Return the cooked shrimp to the skillet. Add soy sauce, oyster sauce, and sesame oil. Stir-fry for another 1-2 minutes to combine.
6. Serve hot, garnished with sesame seeds if desired.

Nutritional Info per Serving:

- Calories: 200
- Protein: 25g
- Carbohydrates: 8g
- Fat: 8g
- Fiber: 3g
- Sugar: 3g

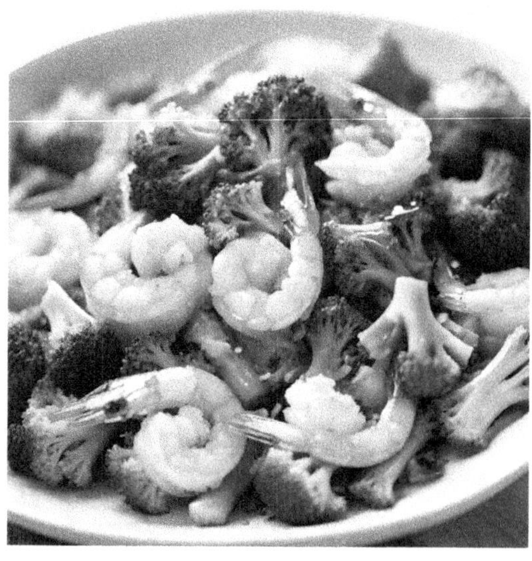

20. Squid with Garlic and Parsley

Servings: 4
Cooking Time: 20 minutes
Ingredients:

- 1 pound squid, cleaned and sliced into rings
- 2 tablespoons olive oil
- 4 cloves garlic, minced
- 1/4 cup chopped fresh parsley
- Salt and pepper to taste
- Lemon wedges for serving

Instructions:

1. Heat olive oil in a large skillet over medium heat.
2. Add minced garlic to the skillet and cook for 1 minute, until fragrant.
3. Add squid rings to the skillet and sauté for 4-5 minutes, until cooked through and opaque.
4. Stir in chopped parsley and season with salt and pepper to taste.
5. Cook for another minute, then remove from heat.
6. Serve hot, with lemon wedges for squeezing over the squid.

Nutritional Info per Serving:

- Calories: 160
- Protein: 20g
- Carbohydrates: 2g
- Fat: 8g
- Fiber: 0g
- Sugar: 0g

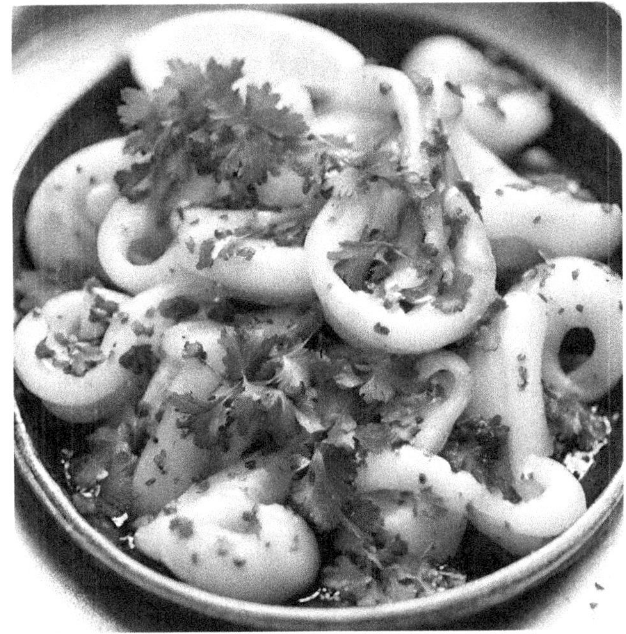

21. Carpaccio of Octopus

Servings: 4

Preparation Time: 20 minutes

Ingredients:

- 1 pound octopus, cooked and thinly sliced
- 2 tablespoons olive oil
- 1 tablespoon lemon juice
- 1 teaspoon capers
- 1 teaspoon chopped fresh parsley
- Salt and pepper to taste
- Arugula leaves for serving

Instructions:

1. Arrange the thinly sliced octopus on a serving platter or individual plates.
2. In a small bowl, whisk together the olive oil, lemon juice, capers, chopped parsley, salt, and pepper to make the dressing.
3. Drizzle the dressing over the sliced octopus.
4. Serve chilled or at room temperature, with arugula leaves on the side.

Nutritional Info per Serving:

- Calories: 180
- Protein: 20g
- Carbohydrates: 2g
- Fat: 10g
- Fiber: 0g
- Sugar: 0g

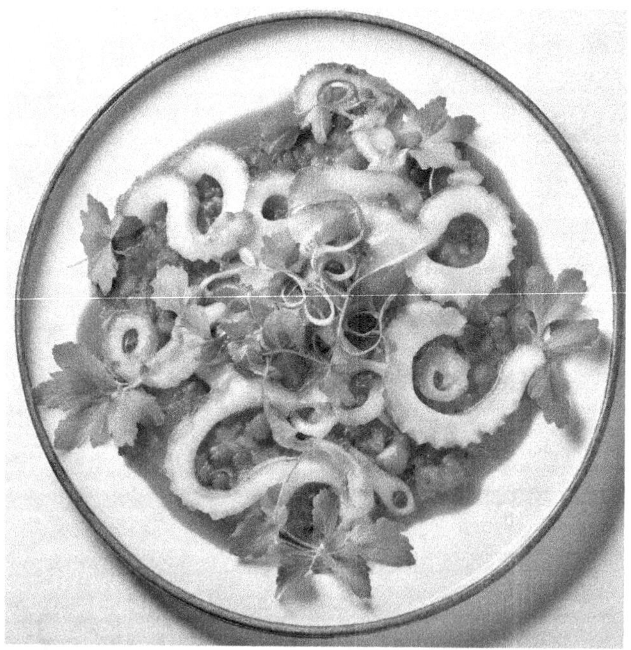

22. Prawn Skewers with Garlic Lime Marinade

Servings: 4
Preparation Time: 20 minutes (plus marinating time)
Cooking Time: 10 minutes
Ingredients:

- 1 pound large prawns, peeled and deveined
- 2 cloves garlic, minced
- 2 tablespoons olive oil
- 2 tablespoons lime juice
- 1 teaspoon lime zest
- 1 teaspoon honey
- 1 teaspoon chopped fresh cilantro
- Salt and pepper to taste

Instructions:

1. In a bowl, combine minced garlic, olive oil, lime juice, lime zest, honey, chopped cilantro, salt, and pepper to make the marinade.
2. Add prawns to the marinade and toss to coat evenly. Cover and refrigerate for at least 30 minutes, or up to 2 hours.
3. Preheat grill to high heat.
4. Thread the marinated prawns onto skewers.
5. Grill prawn skewers for about 4-5 minutes per side, or until prawns are pink and cooked through.
6. Serve hot, garnished with extra cilantro if desired.

Nutritional Info per Serving:

- Calories: 220
- Protein: 24g
- Carbohydrates: 4g
- Fat: 12g
- Fiber: 0g
- Sugar: 2g

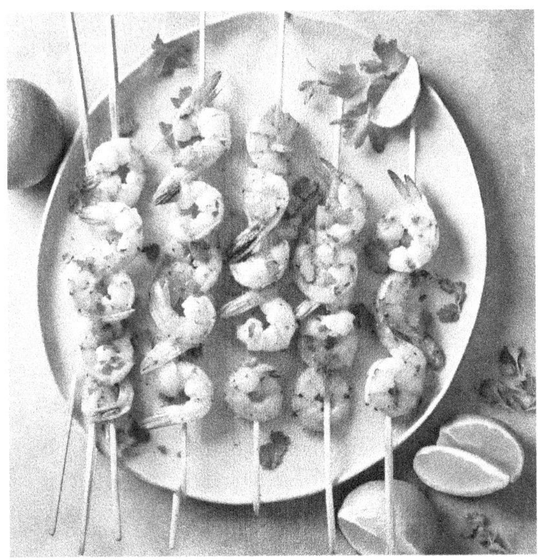

WEEKLY MEAL PLANNER

	BREAKFAST	LUNCH	DINNER	SNACKS
MON				
TUE				
WED				
THU				
FRI				
SAT				
SUN				

Shopping list

Vegetables	Proteins	Healthy Fats

WEEKLY MEAL PLANNER

	BREAKFAST	LUNCH	DINNER	SNACKS
MON				
TUE				
WED				
THU				
FRI				
SAT				
SUN				

Shopping list

Dairy & Alternatives

Miscellaneous

Fruits

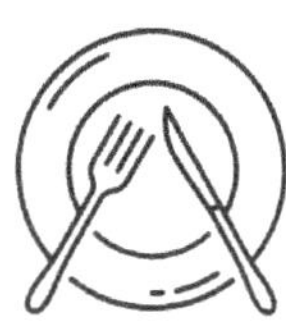# WEEKLY MEAL PLANNER

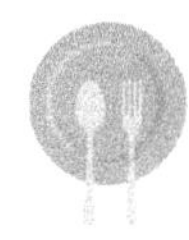

	BREAKFAST	LUNCH	DINNER	SNACKS
MONDAY				
TUESDAY				
WEDNESDAY				
THURSDAY				
FRIDAY				
SATURDAY				
SUNDAY				

What are your main health goals for starting the blood type O diet?

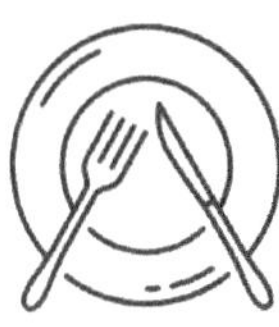

WEEKLY MEAL PLANNER

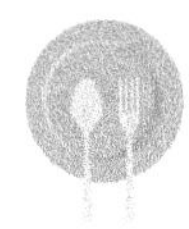

	BREAKFAST	LUNCH	DINNER	SNACKS
MONDAY				
TUESDAY				
WEDNESDAY				
THURSDAY				
FRIDAY				
SATURDAY				
SUNDAY				

List any initial concerns you have about starting the blood type O diet.

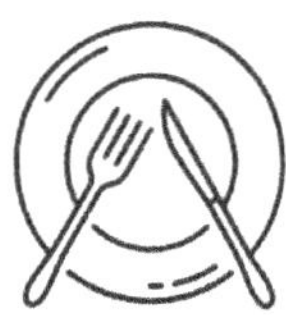

WEEKLY MEAL PLANNER

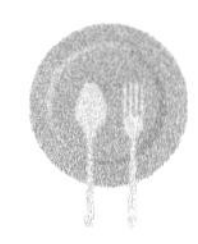

	BREAKFAST	LUNCH	DINNER	SNACKS
MONDAY				
TUESDAY				
WEDNESDAY				
THURSDAY				
FRIDAY				
SATURDAY				
SUNDAY				

What foods from the blood type O diet are you most excited to incorporate into your meals?

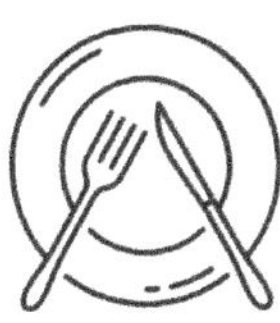 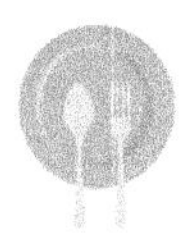

WEEKLY MEAL PLANNER

	BREAKFAST	LUNCH	DINNER	SNACKS
MONDAY				
TUESDAY				
WEDNESDAY				
THURSDAY				
FRIDAY				
SATURDAY				
SUNDAY				

Identify three foods that are discouraged on the blood type O diet that you might miss. How do you plan to manage these changes?

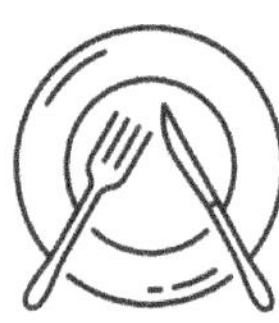# WEEKLY MEAL PLANNER

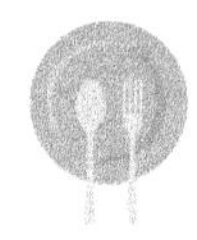

	BREAKFAST	LUNCH	DINNER	SNACKS
MONDAY				
TUESDAY				
WEDNESDAY				
THURSDAY				
FRIDAY				
SATURDAY				
SUNDAY				

How do you feel after eating a meal that is compliant with the blood type O diet? Compare this to how you felt with your previous diet.

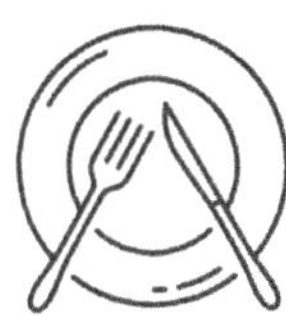# WEEKLY MEAL PLANNER

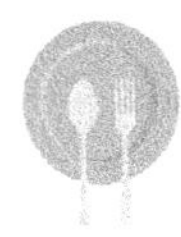

	BREAKFAST	LUNCH	DINNER	SNACKS
MONDAY				
TUESDAY				
WEDNESDAY				
THURSDAY				
FRIDAY				
SATURDAY				
SUNDAY				

Discuss any improvements you've noticed in any pre-existing health conditions.

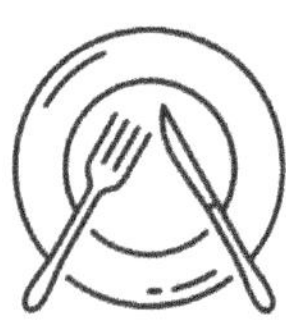

WEEKLY MEAL PLANNER

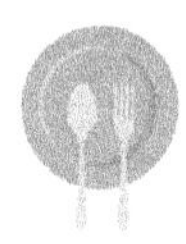

	BREAKFAST	LUNCH	DINNER	SNACKS
MONDAY				
TUESDAY				
WEDNESDAY				
THURSDAY				
FRIDAY				
SATURDAY				
SUNDAY				

Have you experienced any cravings while on the blood type O diet? How have you managed these cravings?

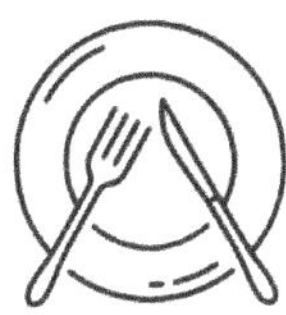 # WEEKLY MEAL PLANNER 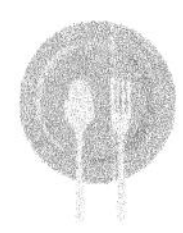

	BREAKFAST	LUNCH	DINNER	SNACKS
MONDAY				
TUESDAY				
WEDNESDAY				
THURSDAY				
FRIDAY				
SATURDAY				
SUNDAY				

What strategies have you found effective for dining out or attending social events while following your diet?

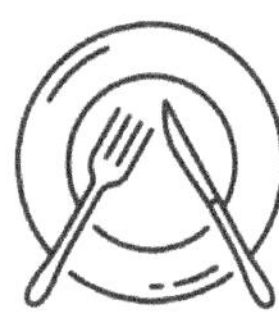

WEEKLY MEAL PLANNER

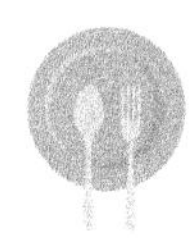

	BREAKFAST	LUNCH	DINNER	SNACKS
MONDAY				
TUESDAY				
WEDNESDAY				
THURSDAY				
FRIDAY				
SATURDAY				
SUNDAY				

Summarize your overall experience this month. What lessons have you learned, and what changes would you like to make moving forward?

WEEKLY MEAL PLANNER

	BREAKFAST	LUNCH	DINNER	SNACKS
MON				
TUE				
WED				
THU				
FRI				
SAT				
SUN				

Shopping list

Vegetables	Proteins	Healthy Fats

WEEKLY MEAL PLANNER

	BREAKFAST	LUNCH	DINNER	SNACKS
MON				
TUE				
WED				
THU				
FRI				
SAT				
SUN				

Shopping list

Dairy & Alternatives

Miscellaneous

Fruits

WEEKLY MEAL PLANNER

	BREAKFAST	LUNCH	DINNER	SNACKS
MON				
TUE				
WED				
THU				
FRI				
SAT				
SUN				

Shopping list

Vegetables

Proteins

Healthy Fats

WEEKLY MEAL PLANNER

	BREAKFAST	LUNCH	DINNER	SNACKS
MON				
TUE				
WED				
THU				
FRI				
SAT				
SUN				

Shopping list

Dairy & Alternatives

Miscellaneous

Fruits

Please Scan this QR Code to Get Your Bonus Content